Virtual Clinical Excursions—O.

for

Murray and McKinney:
Foundations of Maternal-Newborn
and Women's Health Nursing,
6th Edition

Virtual Clinical Excursions—Obstetrics

for

Murray and McKinney:
Foundations of Maternal-Newborn
and Women's Health Nursing,
6th Edition

prepared by

Kelly Ann Crum, RN, MSN
Chair, Department of Nursing
Associate Professor
Maranatha Baptist Bible College
Watertown, Wisconsin

Certified Advanced Facilitator
University of Phoenix
Phoenix, Arizona

software developed by

Wolfsong Informatics, LLC
Tucson, Arizona

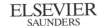
ELSEVIER
SAUNDERS

3251 Riverport Lane
Maryland Heights, Missouri 63043

VIRTUAL CLINICAL EXCURSIONS—OBSTETRICS FOR   ISBN: 978-0-323-22186-3
MURRAY AND MCKINNEY:
FOUNDATIONS OF MATERNAL-NEWBORN AND WOMEN'S HEALTH NURSING
FIFTH EDITION

ISBN: 978-0-323-22186-3

Director, Simulation Solutions: *Jeff Downing*
Content Development Specialist: *Angela Perdue*
Content Coordinator: *Khori Wright*
Senior Project Manager: *Tracey Schriefer*
Publishing Services Manager: *Jeff Patterson*

Printed in the United States of America

Last digit is the print number: 9 8 7 6 5 4 3 2 1

Textbook

Sharon Smith Murray, MSN
Professor Emerita, Health Professions
Golden West College
Huntington Beach, California

Emily Slone McKinney, MSN, RN, C
Nurse Educator and Consultant
Dallas, Texas

Virtual Clinical Excursions Online Reviewers

Kim D. Cooper, MSN, RN
Dean, School of Nursing
Ivy Tech Community College
Terre Haute, Indiana

Kelly Ann Crum, MSN, RN
Chair, Department of Nursing
Associate Professor
Maranatha Baptist Bible College
Watertown, Wisconsin

Certified Advanced Facilitator
University of Phoenix
Phoenix, Arizona

Susan Fertig McDonald, DNP, RN, CS
Clinical Nurse Specialist—Psychiatry
VA San Diego Healthcare System
San Diego, California

Kristin Ulstad Propson, MN, RN
Decorah, Iowa

Jeffrey L. Wagner, PharmD, MPH, RPh, BCPS
Assistant Director
Department of Pharmacy
Texas Children's Hospital
Houston, Texas

Table of Contents
Virtual Clinical Excursions Workbook

Table of Contents
Murray and McKinney:
Foundations of Maternal-Newborn and
Women's Health Nursing, 6th Edition

Getting Started

GETTING SET UP WITH VCE ONLINE ───────────

The product you have purchased is part of the Evolve Learning System. Please read the following information thoroughly to get started.

■ HOW TO ACCESS YOUR VCE RESOURCES ON EVOLVE

There are two ways to access your VCE Resources on Evolve:

1. If your instructor has enrolled you in your VCE Evolve Resources, you will receive an email with your registration details.

2. If your instructor has asked you to self-enroll in your VCE Evolve Resources, he or she will provide you with your Course ID (for example, 1479_jdoe73_0001). You will then need to follow the instructions at https://evolve.elsevier.com/cs/studentEnroll.html.

■ HOW TO ACCESS THE ONLINE VIRTUAL HOSPITAL

The online virtual hospital is available through the Evolve VCE Resources. There is no software to download or install: the online virtual hospital runs within your internet browser, using a pop-up window.

■ TECHNICAL REQUIREMENTS

- Broadband connection (DSL or cable)
- 1024 x 768 screen resolution
- Mozilla Firefox 18.0, Internet Explorer 9.0, Google Chrome, or Safari 5 (or higher)
  Note: Pop-up blocking software/settings must be disabled.
- Adobe Acrobat Reader
- Additional technical requirements available at http://evolvesupport.elsevier.com

■ HOW TO ACCESS THE WORKBOOK

There are two ways to access the workbook portion of *Virtual Clinical Excursions:*

1. Print workbook
2. An electronic version of the workbook, available within the VCE Evolve Resources

■ TECHNICAL SUPPORT

Technical support for *Virtual Clinical Excursions* is available by visiting the Technical Support Center at http://evolvesupport.elsevier.com or by calling 1-800-222-9570 inside the United States and Canada.

Trademarks: Windows® and Macintosh® are registered trademarks.

A QUICK TOUR

Welcome to *Virtual Clinical Excursions—Obstetrics*, a virtual hospital setting in which you can work with multiple complex patient simulations and also learn to access and evaluate the information resources that are essential for high-quality patient care. The virtual hospital, Pacific View Regional Hospital, has realistic architecture and access to patient rooms, a Nurses' Station, and a Medication Room.

■ BEFORE YOU START

Make sure you have your textbook nearby when you use *Virtual Clinical Excursions*. You will want to consult topic areas in your textbook frequently while working with the virtual hospital and workbook.

■ HOW TO SIGN IN

- Enter your name on the Student Nurse identification badge.
- Now choose one of the four periods of care in which to work. In Periods of Care 1 through 3, you can actively engage in patient assessment, entry of data in the electronic patient record (EPR), and medication administration. Period of Care 4 presents the day in review. Click on the appropriate period of care. (For this quick tour, choose **Period of Care 1: 0730-0815**.)
- This takes you to the Patient List screen (see the *How to Select a Patient* section below). Note that the virtual time is provided in the box at the lower left corner of the screen (0730, since we chose Period of Care 1).

Note: If you choose to work during Period of Care 4: 1900-2000, the Patient List screen is skipped since you are not able to visit patients or administer medications during the shift. Instead, you are taken directly to the Nurses' Station, where the records of all the patients on the floor are available for your review.

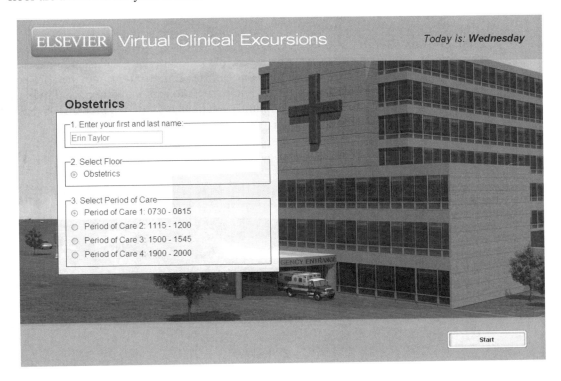

■ PATIENT LIST

Obstetrics Unit

Dorothy Grant (Room 201)
30-week intrauterine pregnancy—A 25-year-old multipara Caucasian female admitted with abdominal trauma following a domestic violence incident. Her complications include preterm labor and extensive social issues such as acquiring safe housing for her family upon discharge.

Stacey Crider (Room 202)
27-week intrauterine pregnancy—A 21-year-old primigravida Native American female admitted for intravenous tocolysis, bacterial vaginosis, and poorly controlled insulin-dependent gestational diabetes. Strained family relationships and social isolation complicate this patient's ability to comply with strict dietary requirements and prenatal care.

Kelly Brady (Room 203)
26-week intrauterine pregnancy—A 35-year-old primigravida Caucasian female urgently admitted for progressive symptoms of preeclampsia. A history of inadequate coping with major life stressors leave her at risk for a recurrence of depression as she faces a diagnosis of HELLP syndrome and the delivery of a severely premature infant.

Maggie Gardner (Room 204)
22-week intrauterine pregnancy—A 41-year-old multigravida African-American female admitted for a high-risk pregnancy evaluation and rule out diagnosis of systemic lupus erythematosus. Coping with chronic pain, fatigue, and a history of multiple miscarriages contribute to an anxiety disorder and the need for social service intervention.

Gabriela Valenzuela (Room 205)
34-week intrauterine pregnancy—A 21-year-old primigravida Hispanic female with a history of mitral valve prolapse admitted for uterine cramping and vaginal bleeding suggestive of placental abruption following an unrestrained motor vehicle accident. Her needs include staff support for an unprepared-for labor and possible preterm birth.

Laura Wilson (Room 206)
37-week intrauterine pregnancy—An 18-year-old primigravida Caucasian female urgently admitted after being found unconscious at home. Her complications include HIV-positive status and chronic polysubstance abuse. Unrealistic expectations of parenthood and living with a chronic illness combined with strained family relations prompt comprehensive social and psychiatric evaluations initiated on the day of simulation.

■ HOW TO SELECT A PATIENT

- You can choose one or more patients to work with from the Patient List by checking the box to the left of the patient name(s). For this quick tour, select Dorothy Grant. (In order to receive a scorecard for a patient, the patient must be selected before proceeding to the Nurses' Station.)
- Click on **Get Report** to the right of the medical records number (MRN) to view a summary of the patient's care during the 12-hour period before your arrival on the unit.
- After reviewing the report, click on **Go to Nurses' Station** in the right lower corner to begin your care. (*Note:* If you have been assigned to care for multiple patients, you can click on **Return to Patient List** to select and review the report for each additional patient before going to the Nurses' Station.)

Note: Even though the Patient List is initially skipped when you sign in to work for Period of Care 4, you can still access this screen if you wish to review the shift report for any of the patients. To do so, simply click on **Patient List** near the top left corner of the Nurses' Station (or click on the clipboard to the left of the Kardex). Then click on **Get Report** for the patient(s) whose care you are reviewing. This may be done during any period of care.

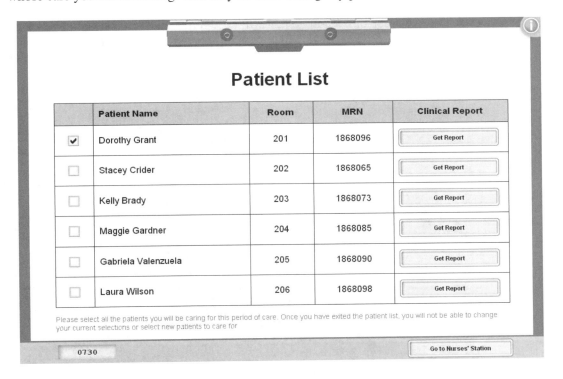

Patient List

	Patient Name	Room	MRN	Clinical Report
☑	Dorothy Grant	201	1868096	Get Report
☐	Stacey Crider	202	1868065	Get Report
☐	Kelly Brady	203	1868073	Get Report
☐	Maggie Gardner	204	1868085	Get Report
☐	Gabriela Valenzuela	205	1868090	Get Report
☐	Laura Wilson	206	1868098	Get Report

Please select all the patients you will be caring for this period of care. Once you have exited the patient list, you will not be able to change your current selections or select new patients to care for

0730   Go to Nurses' Station

■ HOW TO FIND A PATIENT'S RECORDS

NURSES' STATION

Within the Nurses' Station, you will see:

1. A clipboard that contains the patient list for that floor.
2. A chart rack with patient charts labeled by room number, a notebook labeled Kardex, and a notebook labeled MAR (Medication Administration Record).
3. A desktop computer with access to the Electronic Patient Record (EPR).
4. A tool bar across the top of the screen that can also be used to access the Patient List, EPR, Chart, MAR, and Kardex. This tool bar is also accessible from each patient's room.
5. A Drug Guide containing information about the medications you are able to administer to your patients.
6. A Laboratory Guide containing normal value ranges for all laboratory tests you may come across in the virtual patient hospital.
7. A tool bar across the bottom of the screen that can be used to access the Floor Map, patient rooms, Medication Room, and Drug Guide.

As you run your cursor over an item, it will be highlighted. To select, simply click on the item. As you use these resources, you will always be able to return to the Nurses' Station by clicking on the **Return to Nurses' Station** bar located in the right lower corner of your screen.

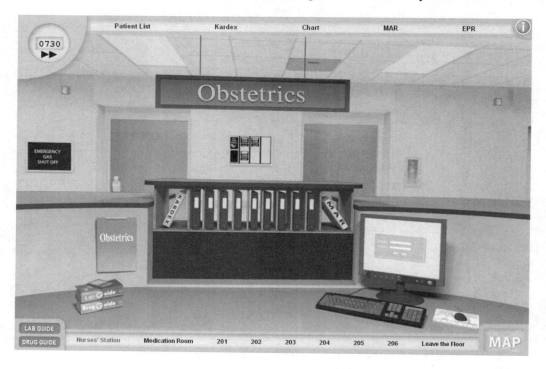

MEDICATION ADMINISTRATION RECORD (MAR)

The MAR icon located on the tool bar at the top of your screen accesses current 24-hour medications for each patient. Click on the icon and the MAR will open. (*Note:* You can also access the MAR by clicking on the MAR notebook on the far right side of the book rack in the center of the screen.) Within the MAR, tabs on the right side of the screen allow you to select patients by room number. Be careful to make sure you select the correct tab number for *your* patient rather than simply reading the first record that appears after the MAR opens. Each MAR sheet lists the following:

- Medications
- Route and dosage of each medication
- Times of administration of each medication

Note: The MAR changes each day. Expired MARs are stored in the patients' charts.

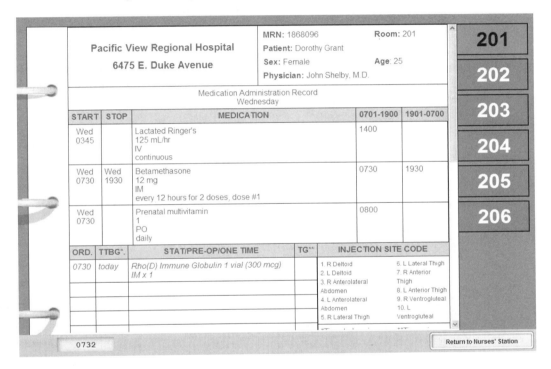

CHARTS

To access patient charts, either click on the **Chart** icon at the top of your screen or anywhere within the chart rack in the center of the Nurses' Station screen. When the close-up view appears, the individual charts are labeled by room number. To open a chart, click on the room number of the patient whose chart you wish to review. The patient's name and allergies will appear on the left side of the screen, along with a list of tabs on the right side of the screen, allowing you to view the following data:

- Allergies
- Physician's Orders
- Physician's Notes
- Nurse's Notes
- Laboratory Reports
- Diagnostic Reports
- Surgical Reports
- Consultations

- Patient Education
- History and Physical
- Nursing Admission
- Expired MARs
- Consents
- Mental Health
- Admissions
- Emergency Department

Information appears in real time. The entries are in reverse chronologic order, so use the down arrow at the right side of each chart page to scroll down to view previous entries. Flip from tab to tab to view multiple data fields or click on **Return to Nurses' Station** in the lower right corner of the screen to exit the chart.

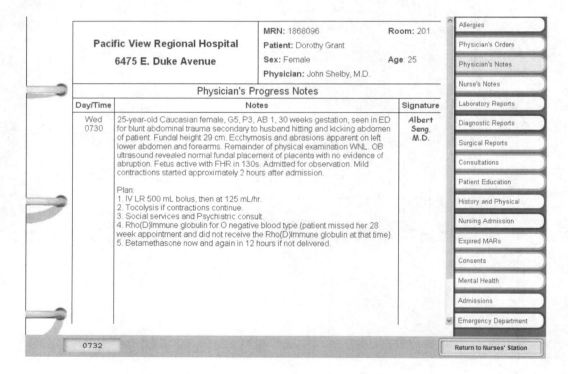

ELECTRONIC PATIENT RECORD (EPR)

The EPR can be accessed from the computer in the Nurses' Station or from the EPR icon located in the tool bar at the top of your screen. To access a patient's EPR:

- Click on either the computer screen or the **EPR** icon.
- Your username and password are automatically filled in.
- Click on **Login** to enter the EPR.
- *Note:* Like the MAR, the EPR is arranged numerically. Thus when you enter, you are initially shown the records of the patient in the lowest room number on the floor. To view the correct data for *your* patient, remember to select the correct room number, using the drop-down menu for the Patient field at the top left corner of the screen.

The EPR used in Pacific View Regional Hospital represents a composite of commercial versions being used in hospitals. You can access the EPR:

- to review existing data for a patient (by room number).
- to enter data you collect while working with a patient.

The EPR is updated daily, so no matter what day or part of a shift you are working, there will be a current EPR with the patient's data from the past days of the current hospital stay. This type of simulated EPR allows you to examine how data for different attributes have changed over time, as well as to examine data for all of a patient's attributes at a particular time. The EPR is fully functional (as it is in a real-life hospital). You can enter such data as blood pressure, breath sounds, and certain treatments. The EPR will not, however, allow you to enter data for a previous time period. Use the arrows at the bottom of the screen to move forward and backward in time.

Patient: 201	Category: Vital Signs				0735	
Name: Dorothy Grant	**Wed 0700**	**Wed 0715**	**Wed 0733**		**Code Meanings**	
PAIN: LOCATION	A			A	Abdomen	
PAIN: RATING	1-2			Ar	Arm	
PAIN: CHARACTERISTICS	I			B	Back	
PAIN: VOCAL CUES				C	Chest	
PAIN: FACIAL CUES				Ft	Foot	
PAIN: BODILY CUES				H	Head	
PAIN: SYSTEM CUES				Hd	Hand	
PAIN: FUNCTIONAL EFFECTS				L	Left	
PAIN: PREDISPOSING FACTORS				Lg	Leg	
PAIN: RELIEVING FACTORS				Lw	Lower	
PCA				N	Neck	
TEMPERATURE (F)	98.2			NN	See Nurses notes	
TEMPERATURE (C)				OS	Operative site	
MODE OF MEASUREMENT	O			Or	See Physicians orders	
SYSTOLIC PRESSURE	126			PN	See Progress notes	
DIASTOLIC PRESSURE	68			R	Right	
BP MODE OF MEASUREMENT	NIBP			Up	Upper	
HEART RATE	70					
RESPIRATORY RATE	18					
SpO2 (%)	96					
BLOOD GLUCOSE						
WEIGHT						
HEIGHT						

Return to Nurses' Station

At the top of the EPR screen, you can choose patients by their room numbers. In addition, you have access to 17 different categories of patient data. To change patients or data categories, click the down arrow to the right of the room number or category.

The categories of patient data in the EPR are as follows:

- Vital Signs
- Respiratory
- Cardiovascular
- Neurologic
- Gastrointestinal
- Excretory
- Musculoskeletal
- Integumentary
- Reproductive
- Psychosocial
- Wounds and Drains
- Activity
- Hygiene and Comfort
- Safety
- Nutrition
- IV
- Intake and Output

Remember, each hospital selects its own codes. The codes used in the EPR at Pacific View Regional Hospital may be different from ones you have seen in your clinical rotations. Take some time to acquaint yourself with the codes. Within the Vital Signs category, click on any item in the left column (e.g., Pain: Characteristics). In the far-right column, you will see a list of code meanings for the possible findings and/or descriptors for that assessment area.

You will use the codes to record the data you collect as you work with patients. Click on the box in the last time column to the right of any item and wait for the code meanings applicable to that entry to appear. Select the appropriate code to describe your assessment findings and type it in the box. (*Note:* If no cursor appears within the box, click on the box again until the blue shading disappears and the blinking cursor appears.) Once the data are typed in this box, they are entered into the patient's record for this period of care only.

To leave the EPR, click on **Exit EPR** in the bottom right corner of the screen.

■ VISITING A PATIENT

From the Nurses' Station, click on the room number of the patient you wish to visit (in the tool bar at the bottom of your screen). Once you are inside the room, you will see a still photo of your patient in the top left corner. To verify that this is the correct patient, click on the **Check Armband** icon to the right of the photo. The patient's identification data will appear. If you click on **Check Allergies** (the next icon to the right), a list of the patient's allergies (if any) will replace the photo.

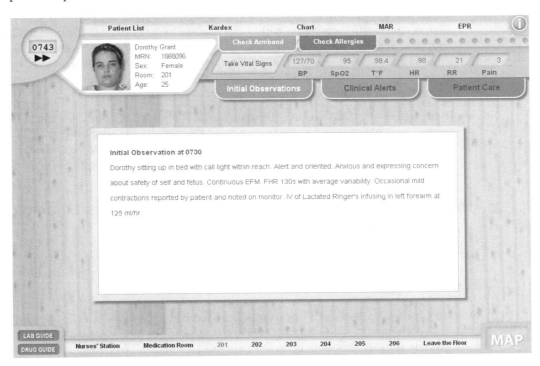

Also located in the patient's room are multiple icons you can use to assess the patient or the patient's medications. A virtual clock is provided in the upper left corner of the room to monitor your progress in real time. (*Note:* The fast-forward icon within the virtual clock will advance the time by 2-minute intervals when clicked.)

- The tool bar across the top of the screen allows you to check the **Patient List**, access the **EPR** to check or enter data, and view the patient's **Chart**, **MAR**, or **Kardex**.

- The **Take Vital Signs** icon allows you to measure the patient's up-to-the-minute blood pressure, oxygen saturation, temperature, heart rate, respiratory rate, and pain level.

- Each time you enter a patient's room, you are given an Initial Observation report to review (in the text box under the patient's photo). These notes are provided to give you a "look" at the patient as if you had just stepped into the room. You can also click on the **Initial Observations** icon to return to this box from other views within the patient's room. To the right of this icon is **Clinical Alerts**, a resource that allows you to make decisions about priority medication interventions based on emerging data collected in real time. Check this screen throughout your period of care to avoid missing critical information related to recently ordered or STAT medications.

- Clicking on **Patient Care** opens up three specific learning environments within the patient room: **Physical Assessment**, **Nurse-Client Interactions**, and **Medication Administration**.

- To perform a **Physical Assessment**, choose a body area (such as **Head & Neck**) from the column of yellow buttons. This activates a list of system subcategories for that body area (e.g., see **Sensory**, **Neurologic**, etc. in the green boxes). After you select the system you wish to evaluate, a brief description of the assessment findings will appear in a box to the right. A still photo provides a "snapshot" of how an assessment of this area might be done or what the finding might look like. For every body area, you can also click on **Equipment** on the right side of the screen.

- To the right of the Physical Assessment icon is **Nurse-Client Interactions**. Clicking on this icon will reveal the times and titles of any videos available for viewing. (*Note:* If the video you wish to see is not listed, this means you have not yet reached the correct virtual time to view that video. Check the virtual clock; you may return to access the video once its designated time has occurred—as long as you do so within the same period of care. Or you can click on the fast-forward icon within the virtual clock to advance the time by 2-minute intervals. You will then need to click again on **Patient Care** and **Nurse-Client Interactions** to refresh the screen.) To view a listed video, click on the white arrow to the right of the video title. Use the control buttons below the video to start, stop, pause, rewind, or fast-forward the action or to mute the sound.

- **Medication Administration** is the pathway that allows you to review and administer medications to a patient after you have prepared them in the Medication Room. This process is also addressed further in the *How to Prepare Medications* section below and in *Medications* in the **Detailed Tour**. For additional hands-on practice, see *Reducing Medication Errors* below the **Quick Tour** and **Detailed Tour** in your resources.

■ HOW TO QUIT, CHANGE PATIENTS, OR CHANGE PERIODS OF CARE

How to Quit: From most screens, you may click the **Leave the Floor** icon on the bottom tool bar to the right of the patient room numbers. (*Note:* From some screens, you will first need to click an **Exit** button or **Return to Nurses' Station** before clicking **Leave the Floor**.) When the Floor Menu appears, click **Exit** to leave the program.

How to Change Patients or Periods of Care: To change patients, simply click on the new patient's room number. (You cannot receive a scorecard for a new patient, however, unless you have already selected that patient on the Patient List screen.) To change to a new period of care or to restart the virtual clock, click on **Leave the Floor** and then on **Restart the Program**.

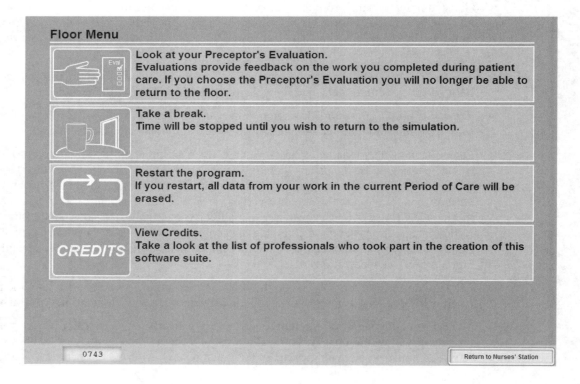

■ HOW TO PREPARE MEDICATIONS

From the Nurses' Station or the patient's room, you can access the Medication Room by clicking on the icon in the tool bar at the bottom of your screen to the left of the patient room numbers.

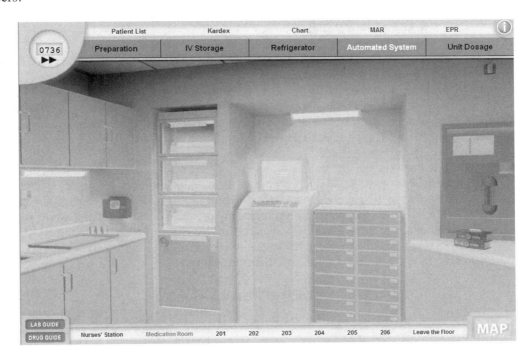

In the Medication Room you have access to the following (from left to right):

- A preparation area is located on the counter under the cabinets. To begin the medication preparation process, click on the tray on the counter or click on the **Preparation** icon at the top of the screen. The next screen leads you through a specific sequence (called the Preparation Wizard) to prepare medications one at a time for administration to a patient. However, no medication has been selected at this time. We will do this while working with a patient in *A Detailed Tour*. To exit this screen, click on **View Medication Room**.

- To the right of the cabinets (and above the refrigerator), IV storage bins are provided. Click on the bins themselves or on the **IV Storage** icon at the top of the screen. The bins are labeled **Microinfusion**, **Small Volume**, and **Large Volume**. Click on an individual bin to see a list of its contents. If you needed to prepare an IV medication at this time, you could click on the medication and its label would appear to the right under the patient's name. (*Note:* You can **Open** and **Close** any medication label by clicking the appropriate icon.) Next, you would click **Put Medication on Tray**. If you ever change your mind or decide that you have put the incorrect medication on the tray, you can reverse your actions by highlighting the medication on the tray and then clicking **Put Medication in Bin**. Click **Close Bin** in the right bottom corner to exit. **View Medication Room** brings you back to a full view of the entire room.

- A refrigerator is located under the IV storage bins to hold any medications that must be stored below room temperature. Click on the refrigerator door or on the **Refrigerator** icon at the top of the screen. Then click on the close-up view of the door to access the medications. When you are finished, click **Close Door** and then **View Medication Room**.

- To prepare controlled substances, click the **Automated System** icon at the top of the screen or click the computer monitor located to the right of the IV storage bins. A login screen will appear; your name and password are automatically filled in. Click **Login**. Select the patient for whom you wish to access medications; then select the correct medication drawer to open (they are stored alphabetically). Click **Open Drawer**, highlight the proper medication, and choose **Put Medication on Tray**. When you are finished, click **Close Drawer** and then **View Medication Room**.

- Next to the Automated System is a set of drawers identified by patient room number. To access these, click on the drawers or on the **Unit Dosage** icon at the top of the screen. This provides a close-up view of the drawers. To open a drawer, click on the room number of the patient you are working with. Next, click on the medication you would like to prepare for the patient, and a label will appear, listing the medication strength, units, and dosage per unit. To exit, click **Close Drawer**; then click **View Medication Room**.

At any time, you can learn about a medication you wish to prepare for a patient by clicking on the **Drug** icon in the bottom left corner of the medication room screen or by clicking the **Drug Guide** book on the counter to the right of the unit dosage drawers. The **Drug Guide** provides information about the medications commonly included in nursing drug handbooks. Nutritional supplements and maintenance intravenous fluid preparations are not included. Highlight a medication in the alphabetical list; relevant information about the drug will appear in the screen below. To exit, click **Return to Medication Room**.

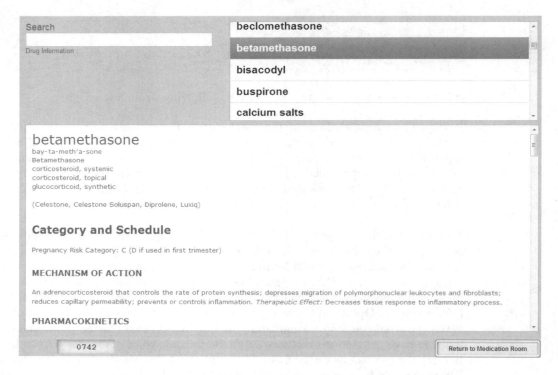

To access the MAR from the Medication Room and to review the medications ordered for a patient, click on the **MAR** icon located in the tool bar at the top of your screen and then click on the correct tab for your patient's room number. You may also click the **Review MAR** icon in the tool bar at the bottom of your screen from inside each medication storage area.

After you have chosen and prepared medications, go to the patient's room to administer them by clicking on the room number in the bottom tool bar. Inside the patient's room, click **Patient Care** and then **Medication Administration** and follow the proper administration sequence.

■ PRECEPTOR'S EVALUATIONS

When you have finished a session, click on **Leave the Floor** to go to the Floor Menu. At this point, you can click on the top icon (**Look at Your Preceptor's Evaluation**) to receive a score-card that provides feedback on the work you completed during patient care.

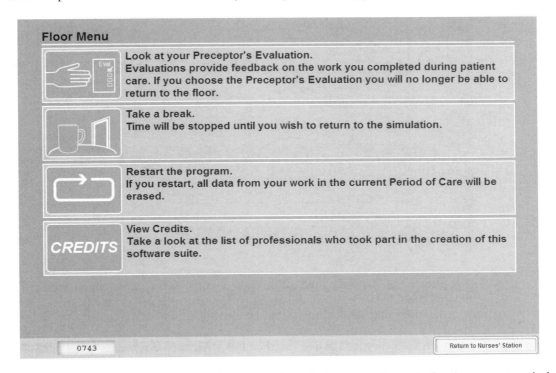

Evaluations are available for each patient you selected when you signed in for the current period of care. Click on the **Medication Scorecard** icon to see an example.

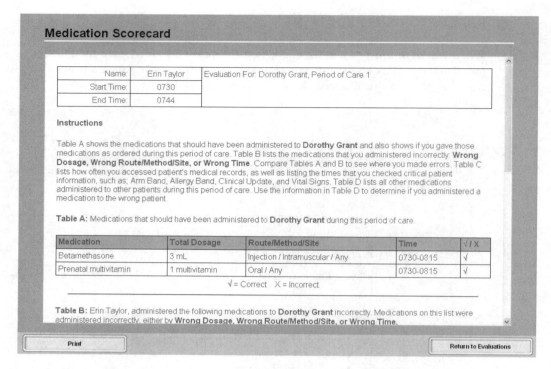

Medication Scorecard

Name:	Erin Taylor	Evaluation For: Dorothy Grant, Period of Care 1
Start Time:	0730	
End Time:	0744	

Instructions

Table A shows the medications that should have been administered to **Dorothy Grant** and also shows if you gave those medications as ordered during this period of care. Table B lists the medications that you administered incorrectly: **Wrong Dosage, Wrong Route/Method/Site, or Wrong Time**. Compare Tables A and B to see where you made errors. Table C lists how often you accessed patient's medical records, as well as listing the times that you checked critical patient information, such as: Arm Band, Allergy Band, Clinical Update, and Vital Signs. Table D lists all other medications administered to other patients during this period of care. Use the information in Table D to determine if you administered a medication to the wrong patient.

Table A: Medications that should have been administered to **Dorothy Grant** during this period of care.

Medication	Total Dosage	Route/Method/Site	Time	√ / X
Betamethasone	3 mL	Injection / Intramuscular / Any	0730-0815	√
Prenatal multivitamin	1 multivitamin	Oral / Any	0730-0815	√

√ = Correct   X = Incorrect

Table B: Erin Taylor, administered the following medications to **Dorothy Grant** incorrectly. Medications on this list were administered incorrectly, either by **Wrong Dosage, Wrong Route/Method/Site, or Wrong Time.**

Print   Return to Evaluations

The scorecard compares the medications you administered to a patient during a period of care with what should have been administered. Table A lists the correct medications. Table B lists any medications that were administered incorrectly.

Remember, not every medication listed on the MAR should necessarily be given. For example, a patient might have an allergy to a drug that was ordered, or a medication might have been improperly transcribed to the MAR. Predetermined medication "errors" embedded within the program challenge you to exercise critical thinking skills and professional judgment when deciding to administer a medication, just as you would in a real hospital. Use all your available resources, such as the patient's chart and the MAR, to make your decision.

Table C lists the resources that were available to assist you in medication administration. It also documents whether and when you accessed these resources. For example, did you check the patient armband or perform a check of vital signs? If so, when?

You can click **Print** to get a copy of this report if needed. When you have finished reviewing the scorecard, click **Return to Evaluations** and then **Return to Menu**.

■ FLOOR MAP

To get a general sense of your location within the hospital, you can click on the **Map** icon found in the lower right corner of most of the screens in the *Virtual Clinical Excursions—Obstetrics* program. (*Note:* If you are following this quick tour step by step, you will need to **Restart the Program** from the Floor Menu, sign in again, and go to the Nurses' Station to access the map.) When you click the **Map** icon, a floor map appears, showing the layout of the floor you are currently on, as well as a directory of the patients and services on that floor. As you move your cursor over the directory list, the location of each room is highlighted on the map (and vice versa). The floor map can be accessed from the Nurses' Station, Medication Room, and each patient's room.

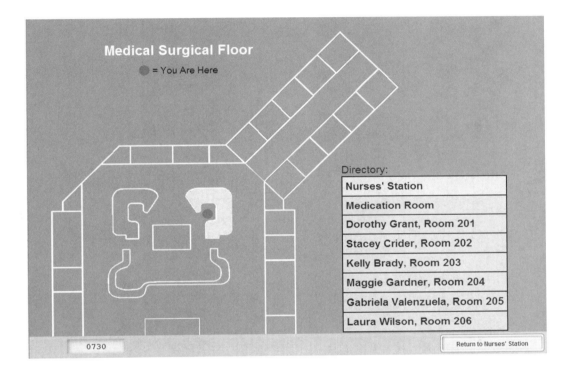

A DETAILED TOUR

If you wish to more thoroughly understand the capabilities of *Virtual Clinical Excursions—Obstetrics*, take a detailed tour by completing the following section. During this tour, we will work with a specific patient to introduce you to all the different components and learning opportunities available within the software.

■ WORKING WITH A PATIENT

Sign in for Period of Care 1 (0730-0815). From the Patient List, select Dorothy Grant in Room 201; however, do not go to the Nurses' Station yet.

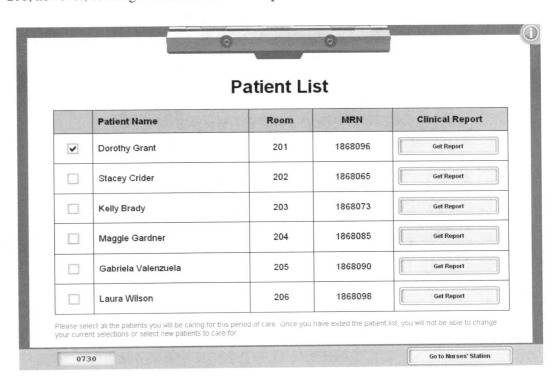

■ REPORT

In hospitals, when one shift ends and another begins, the outgoing nurse who attended a patient will give a verbal and sometimes a written summary of that patient's condition to the incoming nurse who will assume care for the patient. This summary is called a report and is an important source of data to provide an overview of a patient. Your first task is to get the clinical report on Dorothy Grant. To do this, click **Get Report** in the far right column in this patient's row. From a brief review of this summary, identify the problems and areas of concern that you will need to address for this patient.

When you have finished noting any areas of concern, click **Go to Nurses' Station**.

■ CHARTS

You can access Dorothy Grant's chart from the Nurses' Station or from the patient's room (201). From the Nurses' Station, click on the chart rack or on the **Chart** icon in the tool bar at the top of your screen. Next, click on the chart labeled **201** to open the medical record for Dorothy Grant. Click on the **Emergency Department** tab to view a record of why this patient was admitted.

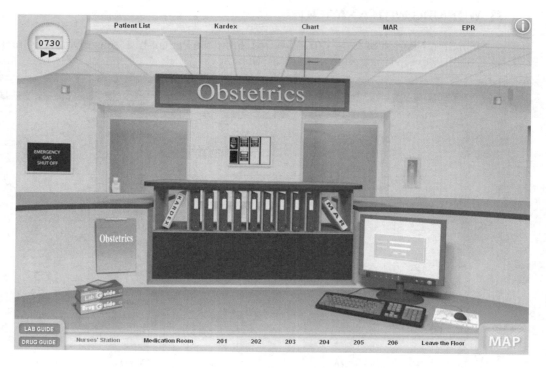

How many days has Dorothy Grant been in the hospital?

What tests were done upon her arrival in the Emergency Department and why?

What was the reason for her admission?

You should also click on **Diagnostic Reports** to learn what additional tests or procedures were performed and when. Finally, review the **Nursing Admission** and **History and Physical** to learn about the health history of this patient. When you are done reviewing the chart, click **Return to Nurses' Station**.

■ MEDICATIONS

Open the Medication Administration Record (MAR) by clicking on the **MAR** icon in the tool bar at the top of your screen. *Remember:* The MAR automatically opens to the first occupied room number on the floor—which is not necessarily your patient's room number! Since you need to access Dorothy Grant's MAR, click on tab **201** (her room number). Always make sure you are giving the *Right Drug to the Right Patient!*

Examine the list of medications ordered for Dorothy Grant. In the table below, list the medications that need to be given during this period of care (0730-0815). For each medication, note the dosage, route, and time to be given.

Time	Medication	Dosage	Route

Click on **Return to Nurses' Station**. Next, click on **201** on the bottom tool bar and then verify that you are indeed in Dorothy Grant's room. Select **Clinical Alerts** (the icon to the right of Initial Observations) to check for any emerging data that might affect your medication administration priorities. Next, go to the patient's chart (click on the **Chart** icon; then click on **201**). When the chart opens, select the **Physician's Orders** tab.

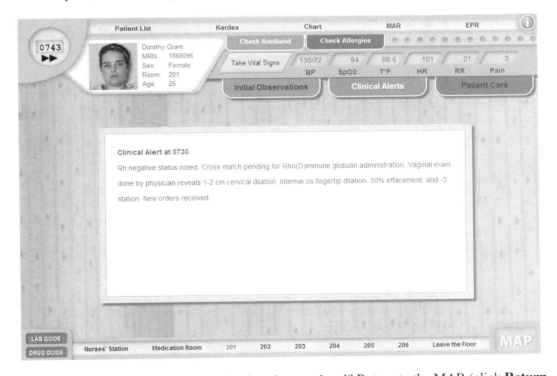

Review the orders. Have any new medications been ordered? Return to the MAR (click **Return to Room 201**; then click **MAR**). Verify that any new medications have been correctly transcribed to the MAR. Mistakes are sometimes made in the transcription process in the hospital setting, and it is sound practice to double-check any new order.

Are there any patient assessments you will need to perform before administering these medications? If so, return to Room 201 and click on **Patient Care** and then **Physical Assessment** to complete those assessments before proceeding.

Now click on the **Medication Room** icon in the tool bar at the bottom of your screen to locate and prepare the medications for Dorothy Grant.

In the Medication Room, you must access the medications for Dorothy Grant from the specific dispensing system in which each medication is stored. Locate each medication that needs to be given in this time period and click on **Put Medication on Tray** as appropriate. (*Hint:* Look in **Unit Dosage** drawer first.) When you are finished, click on **Close Drawer** and then on **View Medication Room**. Now click on the medication tray on the counter on the left side of the medication room screen to begin preparing the medications you have selected. (*Remember:* You can also click **Preparation** in the tool bar at the top of the screen.)

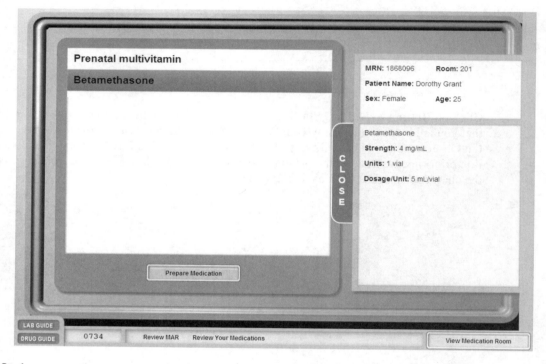

In the preparation area, you should see a list of the medications you put on the tray in the previous steps. Click on the first medication and then click **Prepare**. Follow the onscreen instructions of the Preparation Wizard, providing any data requested. As an example, let's follow the preparation process for betamethasone, one of the medications due to be administered to Dorothy Grant during this period of care. To begin, click on **Betamethasone**; then click **Prepare**. Now work through the Preparation Wizard sequence as detailed below:

> Amount of medication in the ampule: 5 mL.
> Enter the amount of medication you will draw up into a syringe: **3** mL.
> Click **Next**.
> Select the patient you wish to set aside the medication for: **Room 201, Dorothy Grant**.
> Click **Finish**.
> Click **Return to Medication Room**.

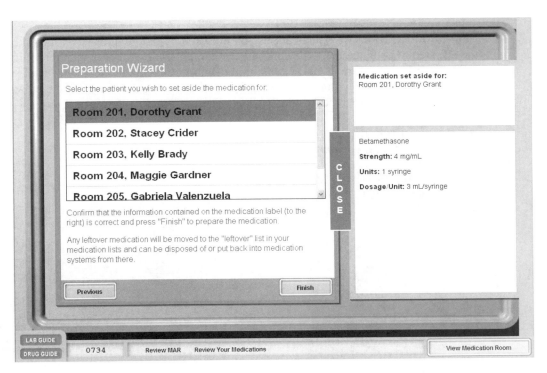

Follow this same basic process for the other medications due to be administered to Dorothy Grant during this period of care. (*Hint:* Look in **IV Storage** and **Automated System**.)

PREPARATION WIZARD EXCEPTIONS

- Some medications in *Virtual Clinical Excursions—Obstetrics* are prepared by the pharmacy (e.g., IV antibiotics) and taken to the patient room as a whole. This is common practice in most hospitals.
- Blood products are not administered by students through the *Virtual Clinical Excursions—Obstetrics* simulations since blood administration follows specific protocols not covered in this program.
- The *Virtual Clinical Excursions—Obstetrics* simulations do not allow for mixing more than one type of medication, such as regular and Lente insulins, in the same syringe. In the clinical setting, when multiple types of insulin are ordered for a patient, the regular insulin is drawn up first, followed by the longer-acting insulin. Insulin is always administered in a special unit-marked syringe.

Now return to Room 201 (click on **201** on the bottom tool bar) to administer Dorothy Grant's medications.

At any time during the medication administration process, you can perform a further review of systems, take vital signs, check information contained within the chart, or verify patient identity and allergies. Inside Dorothy Grant's room, click **Take Vital Signs**. (*Note:* These findings change over time to reflect the temporal changes you would find in a patient similar to Dorothy Grant.)

When you have gathered all the data you need, click on **Patient Care** and then select **Medication Administration**. Any medications you prepared in the previous steps should be listed on the left side of your screen. Let's continue the administration process with the betamethasone ordered for Dorothy Grant. Click to highlight **Betamethasone** in the list of medications. Next, click on the down arrow to the right of **Select** and choose **Administer** from the drop-down menu. This will activate the Administration Wizard. Complete the Wizard sequence as follows:

- Route: **Injection**
- Method: **Intramuscular**
- Site: **Any**
- Click **Administer to Patient** arrow.
- Would you like to document this administration in the MAR? **Yes**
- Click **Finish** arrow.

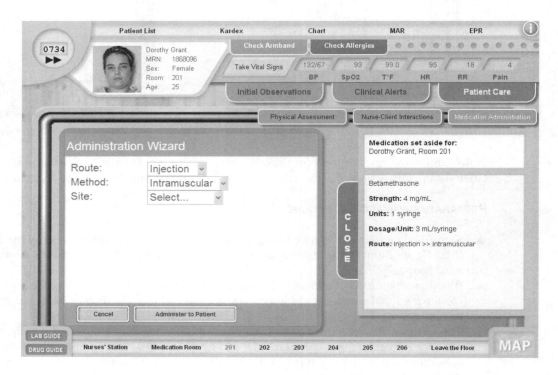

Your selections are recorded by a tracking system and evaluated on a Medication Scorecard stored under Preceptor's Evaluations. This scorecard can be viewed, printed, and given to your instructor. To access the Preceptor's Evaluations, click on **Leave the Floor**. When the Floor Menu appears, select **Look at Your Preceptor's Evaluation**. Then click on **Medication Scorecard** inside the box with Dorothy Grant's name (see example on the following page).

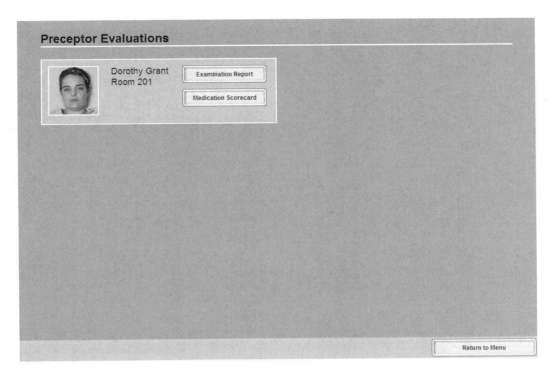

■ MEDICATION SCORECARD

- First, review Table A. Was betamethasone given correctly? Did you give the other medications as ordered?
- Table B shows you which (if any) medications you gave incorrectly.
- Table C addresses the resources used for Dorothy Grant. Did you access the patient's chart, MAR, EPR, or Kardex as needed to make safe medication administration decisions?
- Did you check the patient's armband to verify her identity? Did you check whether your patient had any known allergies to medications? Were vital signs taken?

When you have finished reviewing the scorecard, click **Return to Evaluations** and then **Return to Menu**.

■ VITAL SIGNS

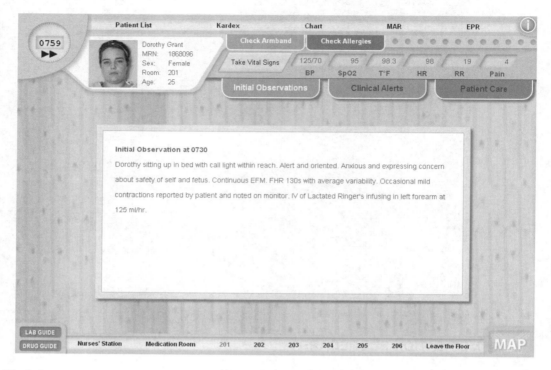

Vital signs, often considered the traditional "signs of life," include body temperature, heart rate, respiratory rate, blood pressure, oxygen saturation of the blood, and pain level.

Inside Dorothy Grant's room, click **Take Vital Signs**. (*Note:* If you are following this detailed tour step by step, you will need to **Restart the Program** from the Floor Menu, sign in again for Period of Care 1, and navigate to Room 201.) Collect vital signs for this patient and record them below. Note the time at which you collected each of these data. (*Remember:* You can take vital signs at any time. The data change over time to reflect the temporal changes you would find in a patient similar to Dorothy Grant.)

Vital Signs	Findings/Time
Blood pressure	
O_2 saturation	
Temperature	
Heart rate	
Respiratory rate	
Pain rating	

After you are done, click on the **EPR** icon located in the tool bar at the top of the screen. Your username and password are automatically provided. Click on **Login** to enter the EPR. To access Dorothy Grant's records, click on the down arrow next to Patient and choose her room number, **201**. Select **Vital Signs** as the category. Next, in the empty time column on the far right, record the vital signs data you just collected in the patient's room. If you need help with this process, refer to the Electronic Patient Record (EPR) section of the Quick Tour. Now compare these findings with the data you collected earlier for this patient's vital signs. Use these earlier findings to establish a baseline for each of the vital signs.

    a.   Are any of the data you collected significantly different from the baseline for a particular vital sign?

        Circle One: Yes   No

    b.   If "Yes," which data are different?

■ PHYSICAL ASSESSMENT

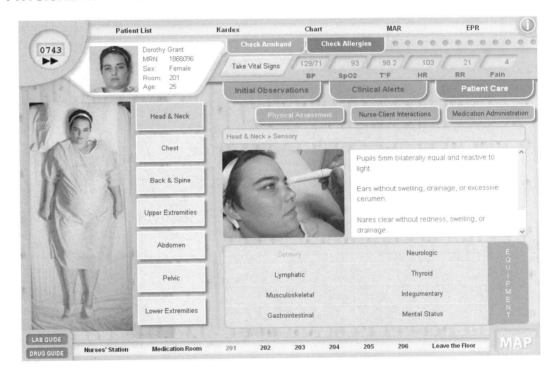

After you have finished examining the EPR for vital signs, click **Exit EPR** to return to Room 201. Click **Patient Care** and then **Physical Assessment**. Think about the information you received in the report at the beginning of this shift, as well as what you may have learned about this patient from the chart. Based on this, what area(s) of examination should you pay most attention to at this time? Is there any equipment you should be monitoring? Conduct a physical assessment of the body areas and systems that you consider priorities for Dorothy Grant. For example, select **Head & Neck**; then click on and assess **Sensory** and **Lymphatic**. Complete any other assessment(s) you think are necessary at this time. In the following table, record the data you collected during this examination.

Area of Examination	Findings
Head & Neck Sensory	
Head & Neck Lymphatic	

After you have finished collecting these data, return to the EPR. Compare the data that were already in the record with those you just collected.

    a.   Are any of the data you collected significantly different from the baselines for this patient?

           Circle One: Yes   No

    b.   If "Yes," which data are different?

■ NURSE-CLIENT INTERACTIONS

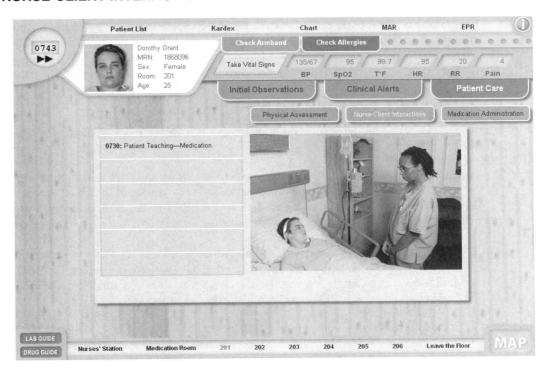

Click on **Patient Care** from inside Dorothy Grant's room (201). Now click on **Nurse-Client Interactions** to access a short video titled **Patient Teaching—Medication**, which is available for viewing at or after 0730 (based on the virtual clock in the upper left corner of your screen; see *Note* below). To begin the video, click on the white arrow next to its title. You will observe a nurse communicating with Dorothy Grant. There are many variations of nursing practice, some exemplifying "best" practice and some not. Note whether the nurse in this interaction displays professional behavior and compassionate care. Are her words congruent with what is going on with the patient? Does this interaction "feel right" to you? If not, how would you handle this situation differently? Explain.

Note: If the video you wish to view is not listed, this means you have not yet reached the correct virtual time to view that video. Check the virtual clock; you may return to access the video once its designated time has occurred—as long as you do so within the same period of care. Or you can click on the fast-forward icon within the virtual clock to advance the time by 2-minute intervals. You will then need to click again on **Patient Care** and **Nurse-Client Interactions** to refresh the screen.

At least one Nurse-Client Interactions video is available during each period of care. Viewing these videos can help you learn more about what is occurring with a patient at a certain time and also prompt you to discern between nurse communications that are ideal and those that need improvement. Compassionate care and the ability to communicate clearly are essential components of delivering quality nursing care, and it is during your clinical time that you will begin to refine these skills.

■ COLLECTING AND EVALUATING DATA

Each of the activities you perform in the Patient Care environment generates a significant amount of assessment data. Remember that after you collect data, you can record your findings in the EPR. You can also review the EPR, patient's chart, videos, and MAR at any time. You will get plenty of practice collecting and then evaluating data in context of the patient's course.

Now, here's an important question for you:

> Did the previous sequence of exercises provide the most efficient way to assess Dorothy Grant?

For example, you went to the patient's room to get vital signs, then back to the EPR to enter data and compare your findings with extant data. Next, you went back to the patient's room to do a physical examination, then again back to the EPR to enter and review data. If this back-and-forth process of data collection and recording seemed inefficient, remember the following:

- Plan all of your nursing activities to maximize efficiency, while at the same time optimizing the quality of patient care. (Think about what data you might need before performing certain tasks. For example, do you need to check a heart rate before administering a cardiac medication or check an IV site before starting an infusion?)

- You collect a tremendous amount of data when you work with a patient. Very few people can accurately remember all these data for more than a few minutes. Develop efficient assessment skills, and record data as soon as possible after collecting them.

- Assessment data are only the starting point for the nursing process.

Make a clear distinction between these first exercises and how you actually provide nursing care. These initial exercises were designed to involve you actively in the use of different software components. This workbook focuses on sensible practices for implementing the nursing process in ways that ensure the highest-quality care of patients.

Most important, remember that a human being changes through time, and that these changes include both the physical and psychosocial facets of a person as a living organism. Think about this for a moment. Some patients may change physically in a very short time (a patient with emerging myocardial infarction) or more slowly (a patient with a chronic illness). Patients' overall physical and psychosocial conditions may improve or deteriorate. They may have effective coping skills and familial support, or they may feel alone and full of despair. In fact, each individual is a complex mix of physical and psychosocial elements, and at least some of these elements usually change through time.

Thus it is crucial that you *DO NOT* think of the nursing process as a simple one-time, five-step procedure consisting of assessment, nursing diagnosis, planning, implementation, and evaluation. Rather, the nursing process should be utilized as a creative and systematic approach to delivering nursing care. Furthermore, because all living organisms are constantly changing, we must apply the nursing process over and over. Each time we follow the nursing process for an individual patient, we refine our understanding of that patient's physical and psychosocial conditions based on collection and analysis of many different types of data. *Virtual Clinical Excursions—Obstetrics* will help you develop both the creativity and the systematic approach needed to become a nurse who is equipped to deliver the highest-quality care to all patients.

REDUCING MEDICATION ERRORS

Earlier in the detailed tour, you learned the basic steps of medication preparation and administration. The following simulations will allow you to practice those skills further—with an increased emphasis on reducing medication errors by using the Medication Scorecard to evaluate your work.

Sign in to work on the Obstetrics Floor at Pacific View Regional Hospital for Period of Care 1. (*Note:* If you are already working with another patient or during another period of care, click on **Leave the Floor** and then **Restart the Program**; then sign in.)

From the Patient List, select Dorothy Grant. Then click on **Go to Nurses' Station**. Complete the following steps to prepare and administer medications to Dorothy Grant.

- Click on **Medication Room** on the tool bar at the bottom of your screen.
- Click on **MAR** and then on tab **201** to determine medications that have been ordered for Dorothy Grant. (*Note:* You may click on **Review MAR** at any time to verify the correct medication order. Always remember to check the patient name on the MAR to make sure you have the correct patient's record. You must click on the correct room number tab within the MAR.) Click on **Return to Medication Room** after reviewing the correct MAR.
- Click on **Unit Dosage** (or on the Unit Dosage cabinet); from the close-up view, click on drawer **201**.
- Select the medications you would like to administer. After each selection, click **Put Medication on Tray**. When you are finished selecting medications, click **Close Drawer** and then **View Medication Room**.
- Click **Automated System** (or on the Automated System unit itself). Click **Login**.
- On the next screen, specify the correct patient and drawer location.
- Select the medication you would like to administer and click **Put Medication on Tray**. Repeat this process if you wish to administer other medications from the Automated System.
- When you are finished, click **Close Drawer** and **View Medication Room**.
- From the Medication Room, click **Preparation** (or on the preparation tray).
- From the list of medications on your tray, highlight the correct medication to administer and click **Prepare**.
- This activates the Preparation Wizard. Supply any requested information; then click **Next**.
- Now select the correct patient to receive this medication and click **Finish**.
- Repeat the previous three steps until all medications that you want to administer are prepared.
- You can click on **Review Your Medications** and then on **Return to Medication Room** when ready. Once you are back in the Medication Room, go directly to Dorothy Grant's room by clicking on **201** at the bottom of the screen.
- Inside the patient's room, administer the medication, utilizing the six rights of medication administration. After you have collected the appropriate assessment data and are ready for administration, click **Patient Care** and then **Medication Administration**. Verify that the correct patient and medication(s) appear in the left-hand window. Highlight the first medication you wish to administer; then click the down arrow next to Select. From the drop-down menu, select **Administer** and complete the Administration Wizard by providing any information requested. When the Wizard stops asking for information, click **Administer to Patient**. Specify **Yes** when asked whether this administration should be recorded in the MAR. Finally, click **Finish**.

■ SELF-EVALUATION

Now let's see how you did during your medication administration!

- Click on **Leave the Floor** at the bottom of your screen. From the Floor Menu, select **Look at Your Preceptor's Evaluation**. Then click **Medication Scorecard**.

The following exercises will help you identify medication errors, investigate possible reasons for these errors, and reduce or prevent medication errors in the future.

1. Start by examining Table A. These are the medications you should have given to Dorothy Grant during this period of care. If each of the medications in Table A has a ✓ by it, then you made no errors. Congratulations!

If any medication has an X by it, then you made one or more medication errors.

Compare Tables A and B to determine which of the following types of errors you made: Wrong Dose, Wrong Route/Method/Site, or Wrong Time. Follow these steps:
   a. Find medications in Table A that were given incorrectly.
   b. Now see if those same medications are in Table B, which shows what you actually administered to Dorothy Grant.
   c. Comparing Tables A and B, match the Strength, Dose, Route/Method/Site, and Time for each medication you administered incorrectly.
   d. Then, using the form below, list the medications given incorrectly and mark the errors you made for each medication.

Medication	Strength	Dosage	Route	Method	Site	Time
	❑	❑	❑	❑	❑	❑
	❑	❑	❑	❑	❑	❑
	❑	❑	❑	❑	❑	❑
	❑	❑	❑	❑	❑	❑

2. To help you reduce future medication errors, consider the following list of possible reasons for errors.

- Did not check drug against MAR for correct medication, correct dose, correct patient, correct route, correct time, correct documentation.
- Did not check drug dose against MAR three times.
- Did not open the unit dose package in the patient's room.
- Did not correctly identify the patient using two identifiers.
- Did not administer the drug on time.
- Did not verify patient allergies.
- Did not check the patient's current condition or vital sign parameters.
- Did not consider why the patient would be receiving this drug.
- Did not question why the drug was in the patient's drawer.
- Did not check the physician's order and/or check with the pharmacist when there was a question about the drug or dose.
- Did not verify that no adverse effects had occurred from a previous dose.

Based on the list of possibilities you just reviewed, determine how you made each error and record the reason in the form below:

Medication	Reason for Error

3. Look again at Table B. Are there medications listed that are not in Table A? If so, you gave a medication to Dorothy Grant that she should not have received. Complete the following exercises to help you understand how such an error might have been made.

a. Perhaps you gave a medication that was on Dorothy Grant's MAR for this period of care, without recognizing that a change had occurred in the patient's condition, which should have caused you to reconsider. Review patient records as necessary and complete the following form:

Medication	Possible Reasons Not to Give This Medication

b. Another possibility is that you gave Dorothy Grant a medication that should have been given at a different time. Check her MAR and complete the form below to determine whether you made a Wrong Time error:

Medication	Given to Dorothy Grant at What Time	Should Have Been Given at What Time

c. Maybe you gave another patient's medication to Dorothy Grant. In this case, you made a Wrong Patient error. Check the MARs of other patients and use the form below to determine whether you made this type of error:

Medication	Given to Dorothy Grant	Should Have Been Given to

4. The Medication Scorecard provides some other interesting sources of information. For example, if there is a medication selected for Dorothy Grant but it was not given to her, there will be an X by that medication in Table A, but it will not appear in Table B. In that case, you might have given this medication to some other patient, which is another type of Wrong Patient error. To investigate further, look at Table D, which lists the medications you gave to other patients. See whether you can find any medications ordered for Dorothy Grant that were given to another patient by mistake. However, before you make any decisions, be sure to cross-check the MAR for other patients because the same medication may have been ordered for multiple patients. Use the following form to record your findings:

Medication	Should Have Been Given to Dorothy Grant	Given by Mistake to

5. Now take some time to review the medication exercises you just completed. Use the form
    below to create an overall analysis of what you have learned. Once again, record each of the
    medication errors you made, including the type of each error. Then, for each error you
    made, indicate specifically what you would do differently to prevent this type of error from
    occurring again.

Medication	Type of Error	Error Prevention Tactic

Submit this form to your instructor if required as a graded assignment, or simply use these
exercises to improve your understanding of medication errors and how to reduce them.

Name: _____   Date: _____

KEY ICONS

The following icons are used throughout this workbook to help you quickly identify particular activities and assignments:

 Indicates a reading assignment—tells you which textbook chapter(s) you should read before starting each lesson

 Indicates a writing activity

 Marks the beginning of an interactive virtual hospital activity—signals you to return to your *Virtual Clinical Excursions* simulation

 Indicates additional virtual hospital activity instructions

 Indicates questions and activities that require you to consult your textbook

 Indicates the approximate time required to complete an exercise

LESSON **1**

Maternity Care Today

 Reading Assignment: Maternity and Women's Health Care Today (Chapter 1)
Ethical, Social, and Legal Issues (Chapter 3)
The Childbearing Family with Special Needs (Chapter 24)

Patients: Dorothy Grant, Room 201
Stacey Crider, Room 202
Kelly Brady, Room 203
Maggie Gardner, Room 204
Gabriela Valenzuela, Room 205
Laura Wilson, Room 206

Objectives:

- Discuss the various types of families, communities, and cultures represented by the different patients.
- Assess and plan care for a patient from a specific culture.
- Explore how your background influences the care that you give to patients who have differing experiences as it relates to community, family, or culture.

Exercise 1

 Virtual Hospital Activity

 15 minutes

Review pages 8-10 of Chapter 1 in your textbook and complete the following exercise regarding family types.

Read question 1 before starting this period of care. Fill in the table as you review each patient's chart.

- Sign in to work at Pacific View Regional Hospital on the Obstetrics Floor for Period of Care 1. (*Note*: If you are already in the virtual hospital from a previous exercise, click on **Leave the Floor** and then **Restart the Program** to get to the sign-in window.)

- From the Patient List, select all the patients to review.
- Click on **Go to Nurses' Station** and then on **Chart**.
- Click on Dorothy Grant's chart (**201**) to begin.
- Click on **Nursing Admission** and find the patient's marital status.
- Click on **History and Physical** and review the Family History section.
- Once you have completed the column for Dorothy Grant in the table below, click on **Return to Nurses' Station** and review Stacey Crider's chart (**202**). Repeat this sequence until you have completed question 1.

1. Under each patient's name below, place an X to indicate that patient's type of family. (*Note:* The answers may be used more than once.)

	Dorothy Grant	Stacey Crider	Kelly Brady	Maggie Gardner	Gabriela Valenzuela	Laura Wilson
Traditional						
Extended						
Single-parent						
Blended						

2. Using what you learned in the patients' charts, along with the information in your textbook, describe the type of family that Gabriela Valenzuela has.

3. Based on the information provided in your textbook, what type of family do you have? Describe how your family fits the description of the family type that you have chosen.

Exercise 2

 Virtual Hospital Activity

 15 minutes

 Just as there are different types of families, there are also various populations of women within every community. To gain a better understanding of this, read pages 8-14, 34-36, and 476-491 in your textbook.

Read question 1 before starting this period of care. Fill in the table as you review each patient's chart.

- Sign in to work at Pacific View Regional Hospital on the Obstetrics Floor for Period of Care 1. (*Note*: If you are already in the virtual hospital from a previous exercise, click on **Leave the Floor** and then **Restart the Program** to get to the sign-in window.)
- From the Patient List, select all six patients.
- Click on **Go to Nurses' Station.**
- Click on **Chart** and then **201** to view Dorothy Grant's chart.
- Click on **Nursing Admission**. (*Hint*: The first four pages of this section will provide information regarding the patient's population.)
- You may also click on **History and Physical** for information to complete the table below.
- Once you have completed Dorothy Grant's column in question 1, click on **Return to Nurses' Station**. Repeat the above steps for each patient.

1. Under each patient's name in the table below, place an X next to each description that applies.

	Dorothy Grant	Stacey Crider	Kelly Brady	Maggie Gardner	Gabriela Valenzuela	Laura Wilson
Adolescent						
Minority						
Older						
Substance abuse						
Homeless						
Immigrant						

2. Laura Wilson is a member of one of the most medically underserved groups. What are two lifestyle choices she has made that represent high-risk behaviors common in this group?

3. List the characteristics of a healthy family.

4. What is the most important factor in regard to disparity in health care outcomes?

5. What are the reasons for high infant mortality rates in the United States despite available care/progress made?

6. What has your experience been with caring for patients with a similar set of circumstances as Maggie Gardner?

7. Based on the information found in the textbook, will you change the way you care for these patients in the future? If so, how? In your community, what resources are available for women who are affected by the issues discussed in this exercise?

Exercise 3

Virtual Hospital Activity

 25 minutes

- Sign in to work at Pacific View Regional Hospital on the Obstetrics Floor for Period of Care 1. (*Note*: If you are already in the virtual hospital from a previous exercise, click on **Leave the Floor** and then **Restart the Program** to get to the sign-in window.)
- From the Patient List, select Stacey Crider and Maggie Gardner.
- Click on **Go to Nurses' Station**.
- Click on **Chart** and then on **202**.
- Click on **Nursing Admission** and review. (*Hint*: See the Role Relationships section.)

  1. Identify a nursing diagnosis that would be appropriate for Stacey Crider and her family.

- Now click on **Return to Nurses' Station** and open Maggie Gardner's chart by clicking on **Chart** and then on **204**.
- Click on **Nursing Admission** and review. (*Hint*: See the Health Promotion section.)

  2. What alternative/complementary therapy does Maggie Gardner use to relieve stomach trouble?

Maggie Gardner and her husband are very religious. According to the textbook, many members of the African-American culture have strong feelings about family, community, and religion. With this information in mind, complete the following activity and questions.

- Click on **Return to Nurses' Station**.
- Click on Room **204** at the bottom of the screen.
- Click on **Patient Care** and then **Nurse-Client Interactions**.
- Select and view the video titled **0730: Communicating Empathy**. (*Note:* Check the virtual clock to see whether enough time has elapsed. You can use the fast-forward feature to advance the time by 2-minute intervals if the video is not yet available. Then click on **Patient Care** and **Nurse-Client Interactions** to refresh the screen.)

3. What does Maggie Gardner's husband verbalize during this interaction that would correlate with a deep sense of religion?

4. Based on interacting with patients in the hospital where you have worked, describe your experience(s) with caring for someone of a different culture. What are some of the ideals that are different from your own? What barriers have you experienced to your care?

5. How comfortable are you with caring for patients from a different culture? Do you find yourself feeling judgmental or attempting to change others? What can you do to learn more about other cultures?

6. What resources are available at your hospital or within your community to enhance your ability to care for a culturally diverse population?

To further explore Jim and Maggie Gardner's spiritual perspective of this event, return to the patient's chart.

 • Click on **Chart** and then on **204**.
• Click on **Consultations** and review the Pastoral Care Spiritual Assessment and the Pastoral Consultation. (*Hint:* Be sure to scroll down to read all the pages in this section.)

7. What does Maggie Gardner "blame" her miscarriages on?

8. Based on your review, what is Maggie Gardner's perception of God?

9. Based on your review of Maggie Gardner's chart during this exercise, what is one underlying theme that you see in the Consultations, Nursing Admission, and History and Physical in regard to religion and this patient's perception of her situation?

LESSON **2** —————————————————————

Nursing Care During Pregnancy

———————————————————————

 Reading Assignment: Physiologic Adaptations to Pregnancy (Chapter 7)
Psychosocial Adaptations to Pregnancy (Chapter 8)

Patients: Maggie Gardner, Room 204
Laura Wilson, Room 206

Objective:

- Identify common physical and psychologic findings associated with each trimester of pregnancy.

Exercise 1

 Virtual Hospital Activity

 20 minutes

Read the section on Confirmation of Pregnancy on pages 82-85 in your textbook.

1. List the presumptive indications of pregnancy identified in your textbook.

 • Sign in to work at Pacific View Regional Hospital on the Obstetrics Floor for Period of Care 1. (*Note*: If you are already in the virtual hospital from a previous exercise, click on **Leave the Floor** and then **Restart the Program** to get to the sign-in window.)
- From the Patient List, select Maggie Gardner.
- Click on **Go to Nurses' Station**.

- Click on **Chart** and then **204**.
- Click on **Nursing Admission**.

2. Place an X beside each of the subjective presumptive indicators of pregnancy that applies to Maggie Gardner, according to the Nursing Admission.

_____ Amenorrhea

_____ Nausea/vomiting

_____ Breast tenderness

_____ Urinary frequency

_____ Fatigue

_____ Quickening

3. Abdominal enlargement is considered a _____ indication of pregnancy.

4. List three positive indications of pregnancy.

→ • Click on **Return to Nurses' Station**.
- Click on Room **204** at the bottom of the screen.
- Click on **Patient Care**.
- Perform a focused physical assessment by clicking on **Abdomen** and then on **Reproductive**.

5. What probable and positive pregnancy indicators are found in the abdominal assessment?

Probable

Positive

Read the sections on Obstetric History and Menstrual History on pages 86-87 in your textbook.

→ • Click on **Chart** and then on **204**.
  • Click on **Nursing Admission**.
  • Scroll to the Pregnancy section.

6. List Maggie Gardner's obstetric history, using the GTPAL format.

7. What is recorded as Maggie Gardner's LMP?

8. Using Nagele's Rule, calculate Maggie Gardner's EDD. Explain how you calculated this date.

Exercise 2

Virtual Hospital Activity

15 minutes

- Sign in to work at Pacific View Regional Hospital on the Obstetrics Floor for Period of Care 4. (*Note*: If you are already in the virtual hospital from a previous exercise, click on **Leave the Floor** and then **Restart the Program** to get to the sign-in window.)
- From the Nurses' Station, click on **Chart** and then on **204** for Maggie Gardner's chart. (*Remember:* You are not able to visit patients or administer medications during Period of Care 4. You are able to review patient records only.)
- Click on **Nursing Admission**.

1. What is Maggie Gardner's gestational age?

2. Maggie Gardner is in the _____ trimester of pregnancy.

3. How would you describe Maggie Gardner's fetus at this gestational age?

- Click on **Return to Nurses' Station**.
- Click on **Chart** and then on **206** for Laura Wilson's chart.
- Click on **Nursing Admission**.

4. What is Laura Wilson's gestational age?

5. Laura Wilson is in the _____ trimester of pregnancy.

Read the section on Maternal Psychological Responses on pages 104-108 in your textbook.

6. Match each of the following behaviors in the pregnant woman with the trimester of pregnancy in which it is most likely to occur.

_____ Woman's primary focus is on herself, not the fetus.   a. First trimester

_____ Woman is ready to have the pregnancy end.   b. Second trimester

_____ Increased pelvic congestion may increase desire   c. Third trimester
for sex.

_____ Emotional lability present.

_____ Woman spends time thinking about the fetus and
daydreaming about what life will be like when it is born.

_____ Ambivalent feelings are common.

_____ Dependence on partner is increased.

_____ General sense of well-being and contentment is common.

_____ "Nesting" behavior occurs.

LESSON 3

Maternal and Fetal Nutrition/Antepartum Fetal Assessment

 Reading Assignment: Nutrition for Childbearing (Chapter 9)
Antepartum Fetal Assessment (Chapter 10)

Patients: Kelly Brady, Room 203
Maggie Gardner, Room 204

Objectives:

- Identify appropriate interventions for maintaining appropriate maternal and fetal nutrition.
- Differentiate among the varying types of assessment techniques that can be used with low-risk and high-risk pregnancy patients.
- Identify various methods of testing that can be used in high-risk pregnancies.

Exercise 1

 Virtual Hospital Activity

20 minutes

- Sign in to work at Pacific View Regional Hospital on the Obstetrics Floor for Period of Care 1. (*Note*: If you are already in the virtual hospital from a previous exercise, click on **Leave the Floor** and then **Restart the Program** to get to the sign-in window.)
- From the Patient List, select Maggie Gardner.
- Click on **Go to Nurses' Station**.
- Click on **Chart** and then on **204**.
- Click on **Laboratory Reports**.

 Review pages 126, 134, and 551 in your textbook for information regarding anemia.

1. What were Maggie Gardner's hemoglobin and hematocrit levels on admission?

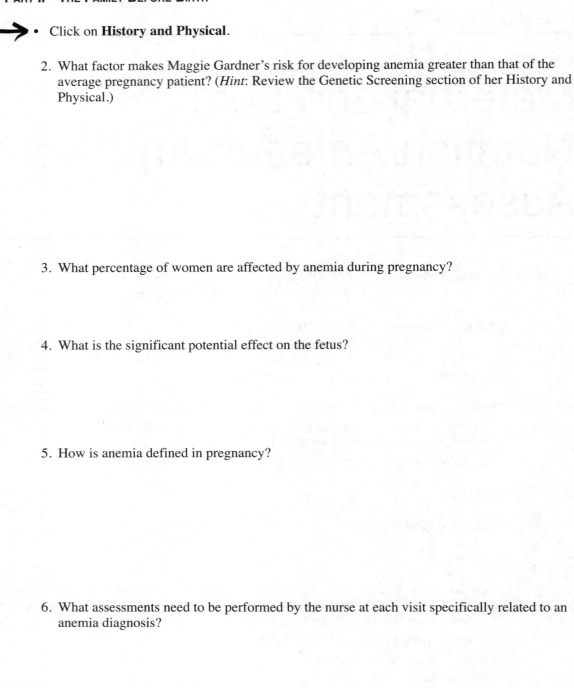

→ • Click on **History and Physical**.

2. What factor makes Maggie Gardner's risk for developing anemia greater than that of the average pregnancy patient? (*Hint*: Review the Genetic Screening section of her History and Physical.)

3. What percentage of women are affected by anemia during pregnancy?

4. What is the significant potential effect on the fetus?

5. How is anemia defined in pregnancy?

6. What assessments need to be performed by the nurse at each visit specifically related to an anemia diagnosis?

 7. According to Table 9-5 in your textbook, what are some good sources of iron that you could instruct Maggie Gardner to add to her diet?

8. Maggie Gardner is not on iron supplementation at this time; however, list three things that you could teach her about iron supplementation. (*Hint*: See pages 126 and 129 in your textbook.)

Exercise 2

 Virtual Hospital Activity

 15 minutes

 Review information regarding ultrasounds on pages 165-168 in your textbook.

1. List three things that ultrasounds are used for during the first trimester.

2. What are two forms of ultrasound? When is each used?

 • Sign in to work at Pacific View Regional Hospital on the Obstetrics Floor for Period of Care 3. (*Note*: If you are already in the virtual hospital from a previous exercise, click on **Leave the Floor** and then **Restart the Program** to get to the sign-in window.)
• From the Patient List, select Maggie Gardner.
• Click on **Go to Nurses' Station**.
• Click on **Chart** and then on **204**.
• Click on **Diagnostic Reports**.

3. What type of ultrasound is Maggie Gardner having?

4. Based on the ultrasound findings, how large is her baby?

5. List three abnormalities found on the ultrasound in regard to the placenta.

6. What is the impression from Maggie Gardner's ultrasound in terms of the fetus and the placenta?

7. What are the recommendations regarding follow-up?

Exercise 3

Virtual Hospital Activity

20 minutes

Biophysical profile is another very important assessment tool used with patients who are experiencing a high-risk pregnancy. Review information regarding biophysical profiles on pages 178-179 in your textbook.

1. What are the five items that are assessed on a biophysical profile?

2. The amount of amniotic fluid provides information about _____
if loss of fluid is not related to premature rupture of membranes.

3. The biophysical profile is an accurate indicator of impending _____.

4. The normal score on a biophysical profile is _____.

➤ • Sign in to work at Pacific View Regional Hospital on the Obstetrics Floor for Period of
Care 3. (*Note*: If you are already in the virtual hospital from a previous exercise, click on
Leave the Floor and then **Restart the Program** to get to the sign-in window.)
• From the Patient List, select Kelly Brady.
• Click on **Go to Nurses' Station**.
• Click on **Chart** and then on **203**.
• Click on **Diagnostic Reports**.

5. What is the estimated gestational age of Kelly Brady's fetus?

6. What is the amniotic fluid index as indicated on the report?

7. How does this correlate with the normal index as listed in the textbook?

8. What is the score on the biophysical profile?

9. What is the major chronic or long-term marker on the biophysical profile? Why?

LESSON 4

Nursing Care During Labor and Birth

👓 **Reading Assignment:** Processes of Birth (Chapter 12)
Nursing Care During Labor and Birth (Chapter 13)
Nursing Care During Obstetric Procedures (Chapter 16)

Patients: Dorothy Grant, Room 201
Gabriela Valenzuela, Room 205
Laura Wilson, Room 206

Objectives:

- Assess and identify signs and symptoms present in each phase of Stage I labor.
- Describe appropriate nursing care for the patient in Stage I labor.
- Identify appropriate nursing assessments immediately following an obstetric procedure.

Exercise 1

Virtual Hospital Activity

20 minutes

- Sign in to work at Pacific View Regional Hospital on the Obstetrics Floor for Period of Care 1. (*Note*: If you are already in the virtual hospital from a previous exercise, click on **Leave the Floor** and then **Restart the Program** to get to the sign-in window.)
- From the Patient List, select Dorothy Grant.
- Click on **Go to Nurses' Station**.
- Click on **Chart** and then **201**.
- Click on **Nurse's Notes**.
- Scroll to the entry for 0730.

1. List the findings from Dorothy Grant's most recent cervical exam.

→ • Click on **Return to Nurses' Station**.
  • Click on **EPR** and **Login**.
  • Select **201** for the patient and **Obstetrics** for the category.

2. At 0700, what was the recorded frequency and duration of Dorothy Grant's contractions?

→ • Now select **Vital Signs** as the category.

3. At 0700, what was Dorothy Grant's recorded pain level?

Read the section on Stages and Phases of Labor on pages 208-214 in your textbook.

4. At this time, which phase of Stage I labor is Dorothy Grant in?

5. For each specific assessment listed below and on the next page, compare the typical findings for latent labor with Dorothy Grant's current condition.

Assessment	Findings for Typical Patient	Findings for Dorothy Grant
Cervical dilation		

Assessment	Findings for Typical Patient	Findings for Dorothy Grant
Contraction frequency		
Contraction duration		
Contraction intensity		

6. List the typical behaviors seen in patients experiencing the latent phase of labor.

➤ • Click on **Exit EPR**.
   • Click on **201** at the bottom of the screen.
   • Click on **Patient Care** and then **Nurse-Client Interactions**.
   • Select and view the video titled **0810: Monitoring/Patient Support**. (*Note:* Check the virtual clock to see whether enough time has elapsed. You can use the fast-forward feature to advance the time by 2-minute intervals if the video is not yet available. Then click on **Patient Care** and **Nurse-Client Interactions** to refresh the screen.)

7. Based on the video interaction, place an X next to each characteristic that is true of Dorothy Grant.

_____ Sociable

_____ Excited

_____ Somewhat anxious

_____ Cooperative

_____ Relieved the pregnancy is about to end

Exercise 2

 Virtual Hospital Activity

 45 minutes

- Sign in to work at Pacific View Regional Hospital on the Obstetrics Floor for Period of Care 2. (*Note*: If you are already in the virtual hospital from a previous exercise, click on **Leave the Floor** and then **Restart the Program** to get to the sign-in window.)
- From the Patient List, select Gabriela Valenzuela.

 Read the section on Application of the Nursing Process: True Labor on pages 233-244 in your textbook.

 • Click on **Go to Nurses' Station**.
- Click on **Chart** and then **205**.
- Click on **Nurse's Notes**.
- Scroll back to the entry for 0800.

1. What was Gabriela Valenzuela's condition at this time? What phase of labor was she experiencing?

 Reread the section on Active Phase on pages 208-214 in your textbook.

2. As Gabriela Valenzuela progresses in labor, which phase will she enter next?

3. List the typical behaviors seen in patients experiencing the active phase of labor.

➤ • Still in the Nurse's Notes, scroll to the entry for 1140.

   4. How is Gabriela Valenzuela tolerating labor at this time? Do you believe she has entered active phase?

   5. How could you determine for certain which phase of labor Gabriela Valenzuela is currently experiencing?

➤ • Click on **Return to Nurses' Station**.
   • Click on **205** at the bottom of the screen.
   • Click on **Patient Care** and then **Nurse-Client Interactions**.
   • Select and view the video titled **1140: Intervention—Bleeding, Comfort**. (*Note:* Check the virtual clock to see whether enough time has elapsed. You can use the fast-forward feature to advance the time by 2-minute intervals if the video is not yet available. Then click on **Patient Care** and **Nurse-Client Interactions** to refresh the screen.)

   6. Based on the video interaction, below and on the next page place an X next to each intervention suggested or implemented by the nurse.

   _____ Assist patient to cope with contractions

   _____ Encourage patient to maintain breathing techniques

   _____ Use comfort measures

   _____ Assist with position changes

   _____ Encourage voluntary muscle relaxation and use of effleurage

   _____ Apply counterpressure to sacrococcygeal area

   _____ Offer encouragement and praise

_____ Keep patient aware of progress

_____ Offer analgesics as ordered

_____ Check bladder; encourage voiding

_____ Give oral care; offer fluids, food, ice chips as ordered

→ • Click on **Patient Care** and then **Nurse-Client Interactions**.

• Select and view the video titled **1155: Evaluation—Comfort Measures**. (*Note:* Check the virtual clock to see whether enough time has elapsed. You can use the fast-forward feature to advance the time by 2-minute intervals if the video is not yet available. Then click on **Patient Care** and **Nurse-Client Interactions** to refresh the screen.)

7. In the list below, place an X next to each intervention suggested or implemented by the nurse and/or Gabriela Valenzuela's husband during the video interaction.

_____ Assist patient to cope with contractions

_____ Encourage patient to maintain breathing techniques

_____ Use comfort measures

_____ Assist with position changes

_____ Encourage voluntary muscle relaxation and use of effleurage

_____ Apply counterpressure to sacrococcygeal area

_____ Offer encouragement and praise

_____ Keep patient aware of progress

_____ Offer analgesics as ordered

_____ Check bladder; encourage voiding

_____ Give oral care; offer fluids, food, ice chips as ordered

Exercise 3

 Virtual Hospital Activity

 30 minutes

• Sign in to work at Pacific View Regional Hospital on the Obstetrics Floor for Period of Care 4. (*Note:* If you are already in the virtual hospital from a previous exercise, click on **Leave the Floor** and then **Restart the Program** to get to the sign-in window.)

• From the Nurses' Station, click on **EPR** and then on **Login**. (*Remember:* You are not able to visit patients or administer medications during Period of Care 4. You are able to review patient records only.)

• Select **201** as the patient's room and **Obstetrics** as the category.

• Scroll to review the entries for Wednesday 1800 and 1815.

1. What are the findings from Dorothy Grant's cervical exam at 1815?

 Consult Table 12-1 on page 211 in your textbook.

2. At this time, which phase of Stage I labor is Dorothy Grant experiencing?

3. Complete the table below, listing typical findings for each assessment in the transition phase of Stage I labor.

Assessment	Typical Findings
Cervical dilation	
Contraction frequency	
Contraction duration	
Contraction intensity	

 Reread the section on Transition Phase on pages 212-213 in your textbook.

4. List the typical behaviors seen in patients experiencing the transition phase of labor.

➤ • Click on **Exit EPR**.
• Click on **Chart** and then on **201** for Dorothy Grant's chart.
• Click on **Nurse's Notes**.
• Read the notes recorded at 1800, 1815, and 1830 on Wednesday.

5. Based on information recorded in the EPR and Nurse's Notes, place an X next to each behavior Dorothy Grant exhibited during the transition phase of labor.

_____ Strong (painful) contractions

_____ Urge to push and bear down during contractions

_____ Leg tremors

_____ Nausea/vomiting

_____ Irritability

_____ Loss of control

Now let's review Laura Wilson's status.

➤ • Click on **Return to Nurses' Station**.
• Click on **EPR** and then on **Login**.
• Select **206** as the patient and **Vital Signs** as the category.

6. Below, record Laura Wilson's assessment findings from 1815 on Wednesday.

Pain location

Pain intensity

➤ • Now select **Obstetrics** as the category.

7. Below, record Laura Wilson's 1830 assessment findings.

Contraction frequency

Contraction duration

➤ • Scroll back through earlier Obstetrics entries until you locate the results of Laura Wilson's most recent cervical exam.

8. When was Laura Wilson's most recent cervical examination performed? What were the results?

 • Click on **Exit EPR**.
  • Click on **Chart** and then on **206** for Laura Wilson's chart.
  • Click **Nurse's Notes**.
  • Scroll to the note for Wednesday 1830.

9. According to this note, what event occurred at 1815?

 Read the section on Amniotomy on pages 304-306 in your textbook.

10. List the immediate nursing actions appropriate for the situation you identified in question 9.

11. According to the Nurse's Notes and your textbook recommendations, did Laura Wilson's nurse handle this situation appropriately? Explain.

12. Based only on the information you have learned about Laura Wilson during this exercise, write the nursing diagnosis that you consider to be of highest priority for her at this time.

13. List several nursing interventions for the nursing diagnosis you wrote in question 12.

Pain Management During Childbirth

 Reading Assignment: Pain Management During Childbirth (Chapter 15)
Nursing Care During Obstetric Procedures (Chapter 16, pages 315-323)

Patients: Kelly Brady, Room 203
Gabriela Valenzuela, Room 205
Laura Wilson, Room 206

Objectives:

• Assess and identify factors that influence pain perception.
• Describe selected nonpharmacologic and pharmacologic measures for pain management during labor and birth.

Exercise 1

 Virtual Hospital Activity

45 minutes

• Sign in to work at Pacific View Regional Hospital on the Obstetrics Floor for Period of Care 1. (*Note:* If you are already in the virtual hospital from a previous exercise, click on **Leave the Floor** and then **Restart the Program** to get to the sign-in window.)
• From the Patient List, select Laura Wilson.
• Click on **Get Report**.

1. What is Laura Wilson's condition when you assume care for her, according to the change-of-shift report?

 • Click on **Go to Nurses' Station**.
• Click on Room **206** at the bottom of the screen.
• Read the **Initial Observations**.

2. What is your impression of Laura Wilson's condition?

 • Click on **Patient Care** and then **Nurse-Client Interactions**.
   • Select and view the video titled **0730: Patient Assessment**. (*Note:* Check the virtual clock to see whether enough time has elapsed. You can use the fast-forward feature to advance the time by 2-minute intervals if the video is not yet available. Then click on **Patient Care** and **Nurse-Client Interactions** to refresh the screen.)

3. What is Laura Wilson's assessment of her current condition? How does this compare with the information you received from the shift report and the Initial Observations summary?

 • Click on **Chart** and then on **206**.
   • Click on **Nursing Admission**.

4. List Laura Wilson's admission diagnoses. (*Hint:* See page 1 of the Nursing Admission form.)

5. What is your perception of Laura Wilson's behavior? What data did you collect during this exercise that led you to this perception?

6. Think about the following questions and then discuss your ideas with your classmates: Do your personal values and beliefs contribute to your perception of Laura Wilson's behavior? If so, how? What nursing interventions might help to overcome your personal biases when dealing with Laura Wilson?

 Read the section on Factors Influencing Perception or Tolerance of Pain—Psychosocial Factors on pages 280-281 in your textbook.

 • Continue reviewing Laura Wilson's **Nursing Admission** as needed to answer question 7.

7. Each woman's pain during childbirth is unique and is influenced by a variety of factors. For each factor listed below and on the next page, explain how that factor influences pain perception (in the middle column). Then, in the right column, list data from Laura Wilson's Nursing Admission that support how that factor might relate to her particular pain perception.

Factor	Typical Effect on Pain Perception	Laura Wilson's Supporting Data
Anxiety		
Culture/ previous experiences with pain		

Factor	Typical Effect on Pain Perception	Laura Wilson's Supporting Data
Preparation for childbirth		
Support system		

Exercise 2

Virtual Hospital Activity

  45 minutes

- Sign in to work at Pacific View Regional Hospital on the Obstetrics Floor for Period of Care 2. (*Note*: If you are already in the virtual hospital from a previous exercise, click on **Leave the Floor** and then **Restart the Program** to get to the sign-in window.)
- From the Patient List, select Gabriela Valenzuela.

 Read the section on Application of Nonpharmacologic Techniques on pages 281-286 in your textbook.

1. Nonclinical touch (such as holding her hand) can communicate _____,

   _____, _____, and _____. When using touch, it is

   important to determine the _____ first. Massage may be very

   effective in _____ and _____.

2. Breathing techniques give a woman a different focus during contractions, interfering with

   _____. Breathing techniques should be used

   _____. The woman should begin with _____

   techniques and progress to more complex ones as _____.

   All breathing patterns begin and end with a _____.

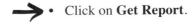 • Click on **Get Report**.

3. Is Gabriela Valenzuela in labor at this time? Give a rationale for your answer.

 • Click on **Go to Nurses' Station**.
  • Click on Room **205** at the bottom of the screen.
  • Click on **Patient Care** and then **Nurse-Client Interactions**.
  • Select and view the video titled **1140: Intervention—Bleeding, Comfort**. (*Note:* Check the virtual clock to see whether enough time has elapsed. You can use the fast-forward feature to advance the time by 2-minute intervals if the video is not yet available. Then click on **Patient Care** and **Nurse-Client Interactions** to refresh the screen.)
  • Click on **Chart** and then **205**.
  • Click on **Nurse's Notes**.
  • Scroll to the entry for 1140 on Wednesday.

4. How is Gabriela Valenzuela tolerating labor at this time?

5. What pain interventions does the nurse implement at this time?

Read about fentanyl in Table 15-1 on page 291 and in the section on Parenteral Analgesia on pages 293-294 in your textbook.

6. What is the action of this drug?

Let's begin the process for preparing and administering Gabriela Valenzuela's fentanyl dose.

➤ • First, click on **Return to Room 205** and then **Medication Room**.
  • Next, click on **MAR** and then on tab **205**.
  • Scroll down to the PRN Medication Administration Record for Wednesday.

7. What is the ordered dose of fentanyl?

➤ • Click on **Return to Medication Room**.
  • Click on **Automated System**.
  • Click on **Login**.
  • In box 1, click on **Gabriela Valenzuela, 205**.
  • In box 2, click on **Automated System Drawer A-F**.
  • Click on **Fentanyl citrate**.
  • Click on **Put Medication on Tray**.
  • Click on **Close Drawer**.
  • Click on **View Medication Room**.
  • Click on **Preparation**.
  • Click on **Prepare** and follow the Preparation Wizard prompts to complete Gabriela Valenzuela's fentanyl dose. When the Wizard stops requesting information, click **Finish**.
  • Click on **Return to Medication Room**.
  • Click on **205** to go to the patient's room.

8. What additional assessments must be completed before you give Gabriela Valenzuela's medication?

9. Why is it important to check Gabriela Valenzuela's respiratory rate before giving the dose of fentanyl?

10. What safety precautions should be in effect for Gabriela Valenzuela after she receives this dose of fentanyl?

 • Click on **Patient Care** and then **Medication Administration**.
  • Click on **Review Your Medications** and verify the accuracy of your preparation. Click **Return to Room 205**.
  • Next, click the down arrow next to **Select** and choose **Administer**.
  • Follow the Administration Wizard prompts to administer Gabriela Valenzuela's fentanyl dose. (*Note:* Click **Yes** when asked whether to document this administration in the MAR.)
  • When the Wizard stops asking questions, click **Finish**.
  • Still in Gabriela Valenzuela's room, click on **Patient Care** and then **Nurse-Client Interactions**.
  • Select and view the video titled **1155: Evaluation—Comfort Measures**. (*Note:* Check the virtual clock to see whether enough time has elapsed. You can use the fast-forward feature to advance the time by 2-minute intervals if the video is not yet available. Then click on **Patient Care** and **Nurse-Client Interactions** to refresh the screen.)

11. How effective were the interventions you identified in question 5?

Read the section on Overcoming Common Problems on pages 285-286 in your textbook.

12. Gabriela Valenzuela is most likely experiencing _____.

    _____ is responsible for the dizziness as well as

    other side effects, including _____,

    _____, and

    _____.

13. What interventions does the nurse suggest to deal with this problem? List other interventions described in your textbook.

 At the end of the 1155 video, Gabriela Valenzuela states that she "doesn't want any needles" in her back. Learn more about this by reading the section on Epidural Block on pages 288-289 in your textbook.

14. What could you tell Gabriela Valenzuela to help her make an informed decision about anesthesia for labor? Below, list advantages and disadvantages of epidural anesthesia.

Advantages	Disadvantages

Before leaving this period of care, let's see how you did preparing and administering the patient's medication.

- Click on **Leave the Floor**.
- Click on **Look at Your Preceptor's Evaluation**.
- Click on **Medication Scorecard** and review the evaluation. How did you do? (*Hint:* For a quick refresher on reading your Medication Scorecard, see the **Getting Started** section of this workbook.)

Exercise 3

Virtual Hospital Activity

  15 minutes

 Read the section on General Anesthesia on pages 295-296 and Cesarean Birth on pages 315-323 in your textbook.

- Sign in to work at Pacific View Regional Hospital on the Obstetrics Floor for Period of Care 4. (*Note*: If you are already in the virtual hospital from a previous exercise, click on **Leave the Floor** and then **Restart the Program** to get to the sign-in window.)
- From the Nurses' Station, click on **Chart** and then on **203** for Kelly Brady's chart. (*Remember:* You are not able to visit patients or administer medications during Period of Care 4. You are able to review patient records only.)
- Click on **Nurse's Notes**.
- Scroll to the entry for 1730 on Wednesday.

1. Why does the anesthesiologist plan to use general anesthesia during Kelly Brady's cesarean section?

2. Why is Kelly Brady upset about receiving general anesthesia for her surgery?

 • Click on **Physician's Orders**.
- Review the entry for Wednesday at 1540.

3. What preoperative medications are ordered for Kelly Brady?

→ • Click on **Return to Nurses' Station**.
   • Click on the **Drug** icon in the lower left corner of your screen to access the Drug Guide.
   • Use the Search box or the scroll bar to read about each of the drugs you listed in question 3.

4. All of these medications are given preoperatively to help prevent aspiration pneumonia. Using information from the Drug Guide and from the section on General Anesthesia in your textbook, match each of the medications below with the description of how it specifically works to prevent aspiration pneumonia.

_____ Sodium citrate/citric acid (Bicitra)   a. Decreases the production of gastric acid

_____ Metoclopramide (Reglan)   b. Prevents nausea and vomiting and accelerates gastric emptying

_____ Ranitidine (Zantac)

c. Neutralizes acidic stomach contents

5. How would you expect general anesthesia to affect Kelly Brady's baby? Why?

LESSON **6** ─────────────────

The Childbearing Family with Special Needs: Adolescent Pregnancy, Delayed Pregnancy, and Substance Abuse

─────────────────────────────────

 Reading Assignment: The Childbearing Family with Special Needs (Chapter 24)

Patients: Kelly Brady, Room 203
                 Laura Wilson, Room 206

Objectives:

- Describe differences in the normal pregnancy changes experienced by adolescent and older mothers.
- Assess and plan care for a substance-abusing woman with a term pregnancy.

Exercise 1

 Virtual Hospital Activity

 20 minutes

Laura Wilson and Kelly Brady represent age extremes among women of childbearing age. Read the section on Adolescent Pregnancy on pages 476-484 in your textbook.

1. In spite of recent decreases, the pregnancy and birth rates for teenagers in the United States

   are _____ than that of European teens. Approximately _____ of

   pregnant teens have had one or more births previously.

• Sign in to work at Pacific View Regional Hospital on the Obstetrics Floor for Period of Care 4. (*Note*: If you are already in the virtual hospital from a previous exercise, click on **Leave the Floor** and then **Restart the Program** to get to the sign-in window.)

• Click on **Chart** and then on **206** for Laura Wilson's chart. (*Remember:* You are not able to visit patients or administer medications during Period of Care 4. You are able to review patient records only.)

• Click on **Nursing Admission**.

2. The table below and on the next page lists several common characteristics of pregnant adolescents, according to your textbook. Based on the information found in Laura Wilson's Nursing Admission, explain how each of these characteristics applies (or does not apply) to her.

Characteristic	Laura Wilson's Supporting Data
Unintended pregnancy	
Inadequate or no prenatal care	
Smoker	
Inadequate weight gain	
Unmarried	

LESSON 6—THE CHILDBEARING FAMILY WITH SPECIAL NEEDS

Characteristic	Laura Wilson's Supporting Data
Not ready for emotional, psychologic, and financial responsibilities of parenthood	
High incidence of STDs	

 Read the section on Delayed Pregnancy on pages 484-485 in your textbook.

- Click on **Return to Nurses' Station**.
- Click on **Chart** and then on **203** for Kelly Brady's chart.
- Click on **Nursing Admission**.

3. The table below and on the next page lists several common characteristics of older primigravidas, according to your textbook. Based on the information found in Kelly Brady's Nursing Admission, explain how each of these characteristics applies (or does not apply) to her.

Characteristic	Kelly Brady's Supporting Data
Pregnancy delayed to pursue a career or for financial reasons	
Decision to become pregnant made after careful thought	

Characteristic	Kelly Brady's Supporting Data
Usually has financial security, a stable relationship, and personal maturity	
Often adopts health-promoting activities	
Receptive to education on child-bearing and/or childrearing topics; likely to seek out information from a variety of sources	
Concerned about complications that may affect the fetus or her own health	

4. Preeclampsia and gestational diabetes occur more frequently in the older gravidas.
   a. True
   b. False

5. The risk for multiple birth (twins, triplets, etc.) decreases with advanced maternal age.
   a. True
   b. False

Exercise 2

Virtual Hospital Activity

20 minutes

- Sign in to work at Pacific View Regional Hospital on the Obstetrics Floor for Period of Care 2. (*Note*: If you are already in the virtual hospital from a previous exercise, click on **Leave the Floor** and then **Restart the Program** to get to the sign-in window.)
- From the Patient List, select Laura Wilson.
- Click on **Go to Nurses' Station**.
- Click on **Chart** and then **206**.
- Click on **Nursing Admission**.

1. Complete the table below by documenting Laura Wilson's use of alcohol and recreational drugs, based on your review of the Nursing Admission.

Substance	Reported Use
Tobacco	
Alcohol	
Marijuana	
Crack cocaine	

 Read about tobacco, alcohol, marijuana, and cocaine in the Substance Abuse section on pages 486-491 in your textbook.

2. For each pregnancy-related risk listed in the table below and on the next page, place an X under the substance(s) thought to be associated with that risk. (*Hint:* Consult Table 24-2 on page 486 in your textbook.)

Pregnancy-Related Risk	Tobacco	Alcohol	Marijuana	Cocaine
Spontaneous abortion				
Premature rupture of membranes				
Preterm labor				

Pregnancy-Related Risk	Tobacco	Alcohol	Marijuana	Cocaine
Decreased placental perfusion				
Abruptio placentae				
Inadequate maternal weight gain				
Anemia				
Hypertension				
Fetal alcohol syndrome (FAS)				
Fetal alcohol effects (FAE)				
Fetal demise				
Congenital abnormalities				
Intrauterine growth restriction (IUGR) or low birth rate (LBW)				

- Click on **Return to Nurses' Station**.
- Click on **206** at the bottom of the screen.
- Click on **Patient Care** and then on **Nurse-Client Interactions**.
- Select and view the video titled **1115: Teaching—Effects of Drug Use**. (*Note:* Check the virtual clock to see whether enough time has elapsed. You can use the fast-forward feature to advance the time by 2-minute intervals if the video is not yet available. Then click on **Patient Care** and **Nurse-Client Interactions** to refresh the screen.)

3. Does Laura Wilson consider herself to be addicted? Support your answer with comments from the video.

4. How does Laura Wilson think her drug use will affect her baby?

5. According to the nurse in the video, how might Laura Wilson's drug use affect the baby?

Read the section on Interventions on pages 488-491 in your textbook.

6. Assume that you are the nurse caring for Laura Wilson today. Which interventions would be most appropriate to deal with her drug use at this time?

_____ Display a nonjudgmental attitude, as well as genuine interest and concern.

_____ Urge her to begin a drug treatment program today.

_____ Explain to Laura Wilson that she may lose custody of her baby if her drug use continues.

_____ Involve other members of the health care team in Laura Wilson's care.

7. Explain your choice(s) in question 6.

LESSON 7

The Childbearing Family with Special Needs: Perinatal Loss

 Reading Assignment: The Childbearing Family with Special Needs (Chapter 24)

Patient: Maggie Gardner, Room 204

Objectives:

- Identify the various types of loss as they relate to a pregnancy.
- Describe the stages and phases of the grieving process.
- Identify various methods of coping exhibited by patients who have experienced the loss of a newborn.

Exercise 1

 Clinical Preparation: Writing Activity

 15 minutes

Review pages 491-496 in your textbook.

1. Parents may grieve not only the death of a newborn but also the birth of a baby with an

   _____.

2. At what other times might couples grieve a loss related to pregnancy?

89

3. With multifetal pregnancy loss and a concurrent survival of one or more of the infants, what emotions do these parents experience? How does this affect the grieving process?

4. What potential problem may affect a pregnant woman who has experienced a previous pregnancy loss?

5. Ectopic pregnancy is more common in women over 35, increasing the impact if the woman

   has experienced _____.

6. All women and men who undergo a loss receive the support that they need.
   a. True
   b. False

Exercise 2

 Virtual Hospital Activity

 15 minutes

- Sign in to work at Pacific View Regional Hospital on the Obstetrics Floor for Period of Care 4. (*Note*: If you are already in the virtual hospital from a previous exercise, click on **Leave the Floor** and then **Restart the Program** to get to the sign-in window.)
- Click on **Chart** and then on **204** for Maggie Gardner's chart. (*Remember:* You are not able to visit patients or administer medications during Period of Care 4. You are able to review patient records only.)
- Review the **History and Physical**.

1. How many losses related to pregnancy has Maggie Gardner experienced?

• Click on the **Nursing Admission**.

2. What is the first evidence you find that Maggie Gardner's previous losses are affecting her current pregnancy and care? (*Hint*: Review the first five sections.)

 • Click on the **Consultations** tab.

3. To what does Maggie Gardner attribute her inability to have a child?

4. List three therapeutic measures the chaplain can use to assist her through these feelings as part of her grieving process.

5. What did the chaplain accomplish during his time with Maggie Gardner?

Exercise 3

 Virtual Hospital Activity

 20 minutes

 Review pages 493-496 in your textbook.

1. What is an appropriate nursing diagnosis related to grief over a newborn loss or anomaly?

2. What is the typical initial response to such a loss?

3. During assessment, how does a nurse know that the grieving process has been successful in the initial phase?

4. List some subtle cues that may indicate further need for investigation during the grieving process.

5. Acknowledging the infant is crucial in helping the parents work through their loss. What are the rights of the baby that may help the parents through the grieving process?

6. What is the nurse's role in assisting the parents and other family members during this time?

7. Based on the information you have read in the textbook regarding the grieving process, let's explore your personal experiences. Have you ever suffered a loss or taken care of a patient who had just experienced a loss? What emotions did you experience or perceive from that patient? What responses did you communicate to them? Were they therapeutic? How might you have handled this experience differently?

 • Sign in to work at Pacific View Regional Hospital on the Obstetrics Floor for Period of Care 4. (*Note:* If you are already in the virtual hospital from a previous exercise, click on **Leave the Floor** and then **Restart the Program** to get to the sign-in window.)
  • Click on **Chart** and then on **204** for Maggie Gardner's chart. (*Remember:* You are not able to visit patients or administer medications during Period of Care 4. You are able to review patient records only.)
  • Review the **History and Physical**.

8. You have now reviewed Maggie Gardner's History and Physical and compared her information with your textbook's discussion of what happens during the reorganization phase. What correlation do you see?

• Click on **Consultations**.
• Scroll down to review the Pastoral Care Spiritual Assessment.

9. Culture and religion play very large roles in how individuals handle a loss. How has Maggie Gardner handled her losses? (*Hint*: See the Spirituality/Faith Factors section of this consult.)

LESSON 8

The Childbearing Family with Special Needs: Intimate Partner Violence

---

 Reading Assignment: The Childbearing Family with Special Needs (Chapter 24)

Patient: Dorothy Grant, Room 201

Objectives:

- Discuss the statistics related to intimate partner violence (IPV).
- List characteristics of battered women.
- Explore the myths and facts regarding IPV.
- Identify the nurse's role in regard to battered women or those affected by IPV.

Exercise 1

 Clinical Preparation: Writing Activity

 20 minutes

 To answer questions 1 through 7, review the information on pages 497-502 of the textbook. (*Note:* Intimate Partner Violence will be abbreviated IPV.)

1. Match the following descriptions of abuse with the statistics that apply.

_____	Percentage of abused women who abuse their children	a. 35.6%
		b. up to 20%
_____	Percentage of women who are victims of severe IPV	c. 33% to 77%
_____	Percentage of women who experience physical forms of IPV at some point in life	d. 27%
		e. 24.3%
_____	Percentage of women's homes in which the children are also injured	
_____	Estimated percentage of women who are victims of IPV during pregnancy	

Historically, women have often been treated inhumanely. This continues even today. Based on information from the textbook, please select true or false for each of the following questions.

2. The postpartum period is the time of greatest risk for women to be abused by their partners.
   a. True
   b. False

3. Physical abuse during pregnancy may result in fetal death.
   a. True
   b. False

4. Substance abuse is often associated with physical abuse.
   a. True
   b. False

5. Physical violence is limited to hitting and slapping.
   a. True
   b. False

6. Children who are abused are more likely to become abusive adults compared with children who have never been abused.
   a. True
   b. False

Exercise 2

 Virtual Hospital Activity

 15 minutes

- Sign in to work at Pacific View Regional Hospital on the Obstetrics Floor for Period of Care 1. (*Note*: If you are already in the virtual hospital from a previous exercise, click on **Leave the Floor** and then **Restart the Program** to get to the sign-in window.)
- From the Patient List, select Dorothy Grant.
- Click on **Go to Nurses' Station**.
- Click on **Chart** and then **201**.
- Click on **Nursing Admission**.

In addition to reading about Dorothy Grant's perspective on the abusive relationship she has experienced, review the characteristics of battered women found on pages 498-501 in the textbook.

1. What is the reality of Dorothy Grant's situation? How does that correlate with the textbook reading?

 • Click on **Return to Nurses' Station**.
 • Click on Room **201** at the bottom of the screen.
 • Click on **Patient Care** and then **Nurse-Client Interactions**.
 • Select and view the video titled **0810: Monitoring/Patient Support**. (*Note:* Check the virtual clock to see whether enough time has elapsed. You can use the fast-forward feature to advance the time by 2-minute intervals if the video is not yet available. Then click on **Patient Care** and **Nurse-Client Interactions** to refresh the screen.)

2. In the video interaction, what does Dorothy Grant say she should do to help prevent the violence?

3. In the video, what are the patient's current concerns?

Exercise 3

 Virtual Hospital Activity

 15 minutes

 • Sign in to work at Pacific View Regional Hospital on the Obstetrics Floor for Period of Care 3. (*Note*: If you are already in the virtual hospital from a previous exercise, click on **Leave the Floor** and then **Restart the Program** to get to the sign-in window.)
 • From the Patient List, select Dorothy Grant.
 • Click on **Go to Nurses' Station**.
 • Click on **Chart** and then **201**.
 • Click on **Consultations** and review the Psychiatric Consult and the Social Work Consult.

Review the information regarding the myths and facts about intimate partner violence on pages 498-499 in the textbook. Based on that information and your review of Dorothy Grant's chart, answer the following questions.

1. Dorothy Grant stays in the relationship because of _____ and

   _____.

2. The percentage of women who are battered during pregnancy is _____.

3. Based on the information provided, in what phase of the abuse cycle is Dorothy Grant?

4. According to the consults, Dorothy Grant has several options. What are some of the options that the social worker and psychiatric heath care provider can offer her or assist her with?

5. Battering often escalates or begins during pregnancy.
   a. True
   b. False

6. Dorothy Grant's husband blames her for the pregnancy.
   a. True
   b. False

7. Dorothy Grant stays in the relationship because she likes to be beaten and deliberately provokes the attacks on occasion.
   a. True
   b. False

Exercise 4

 Virtual Hospital Activity

 15 minutes

- Sign in to work at Pacific View Regional Hospital on the Obstetrics Floor for Period of Care 4. (*Note:* If you are already in the virtual hospital from a previous exercise, click on **Leave the Floor** and then **Restart the Program** to get to the sign-in window.)
- From the Nurses' Station, click on **Kardex** and then on tab **201** to review Dorothy Grant's record. (*Remember:* You are not able to visit patients or administer medications during Period of Care 4. You are able to review patient records only.)

1. What action was initiated on Wednesday to protect Dorothy Grant from her husband?

2. What care plan diagnoses are appropriate for this patient's current life situation?

3. What other disciplines have been contacted or consulted that will ensure continuity of care for Dorothy Grant as it relates to her abuse?

In your textbook, review pages 499-501 to assist in answering the following questions.

4. As a nurse caring for Dorothy Grant, what is your responsibility for reporting IPV?

5. What are the reporting requirements of the state in which you practice?

6. What are the resources available in your area for women who have experienced intimate partner violence?

9

Complications of Pregnancy: Hypertensive Disorders of Pregnancy

 Reading Assignment: Complications of Pregnancy (Chapter 25, pages 519-530)

Patient: Kelly Brady, Room 203

Objectives:

- Assess and identify signs and symptoms present in the patient with severe preeclampsia.
- Explain how common signs and symptoms present in the patient with severe preeclampsia relate to the underlying pathophysiology of this disease.
- Identify the patient who has developed HELLP syndrome.
- Describe routine nursing care for the patient with severe preeclampsia who is receiving magnesium sulfate.

Exercise 1

 Virtual Hospital Activity

20 minutes

- Sign in to work at Pacific View Regional Hospital on the Obstetrics Floor for Period of Care 3. (*Note*: If you are already in the virtual hospital from a previous exercise, click on **Leave the Floor** and then **Restart the Program** to get to the sign-in window.)
- From the Patient List, select Kelly Brady.
- Click on **Go to Nurses' Station**.
- Click on **Chart** and then **203**.
- Click on **History and Physical**.

1. What was Kelly Brady's admission diagnosis?

2. Use the History and Physical and Table 25-2 on page 523 in your textbook to complete the table below.

Sign/Symptom	Mild Preeclampsia	Severe Preeclampsia	Kelly Brady on Admission
Systolic blood pressure			
Diastolic blood pressure			
Proteinuria			
Headache (severe, unrelenting)			
Visual disturbances (spots, temporary blindness, photophobia)			
Right upper quadrant or epigastric pain			

• Click on **Physician's Orders** and find the admitting physician's orders on Tuesday at 1030.

3. What tests/procedures did Kelly Brady's physician order to confirm the diagnosis of severe preeclampsia?

 • Click on **Physician's Notes**.
  • Scroll to the note for Wednesday 0730.

4. What subjective and objective data recorded here would support the diagnosis of severe preeclampsia?

Kelly Brady's 24-hour urine collection was completed and sent to the lab at 1230.

 • Click on **Laboratory Reports**.
  • Scroll to find the Wednesday 1230 results.

5. Below, record the results of Kelly Brady's 24-hour urine collection.

6. Now list all the data you have collected during this exercise that confirm Kelly Brady's diagnosis of severe preeclampsia.

Exercise 2

Virtual Hospital Activity

20 minutes

- Sign in to work at Pacific View Regional Hospital on the Obstetrics Floor for Period of Care 1. (*Note*: If you are already in the virtual hospital from a previous exercise, click on **Leave the Floor** and then **Restart the Program** to get to the sign-in window.)
- From the Patient List, select Kelly Brady.
- Click on **Go to Nurses' Station**.
- Click on **203** at the bottom of the screen.
- Click on **Take Vital Signs**.

1. Record Kelly Brady's vital signs for 0730 below.

- Now click on **Patient Care**. To perform a focused physical assessment, select the various body areas (yellow boxes) and system subcategories (green boxes) as listed in question 2.

2. Record your findings from the focused assessment of Kelly Brady in the table below and on the next page.

Assessment Area	Kelly Brady's Findings
Head & Neck Sensory	
Neurologic	
Chest Respiratory	

Assessment Area	Kelly Brady's Findings
Abdomen Gastrointestinal	
Lower Extremities Neurologic	

 Read pages 520-521 in your textbook; then answer questions 3 and 4.

3. Preeclampsia is caused by _____.

4. Match each of the signs or symptoms below with the preeclampsia-associated pathology it indicates. (*Note:* Some letters will be used more than once.)

_____ Blurred vision/blind spots   a. Generalized vasoconstriction

_____ Headache   b. Glomerular damage

_____ Epigastric or right upper quadrant   c. Vasoconstriction of cerebral vessels;
        abdominal pain   arterial vasospasm

_____ 4+ reflexes/clonus   d. Hepatic edema; hemorrhagic necrosis

_____ Elevated blood pressure

_____ Proteinuria/oliguria

Exercise 3

 Virtual Hospital Activity

 30 minutes

- Sign in to work at Pacific View Regional Hospital on the Obstetrics Floor for Period of Care 3. (*Note*: If you are already in the virtual hospital from a previous exercise, click on **Leave the Floor** and then **Restart the Program** to get to the sign-in window.)
- From the Patient List, select Kelly Brady.
- Click on **Go to Nurses' Station**.

Read about HELLP syndrome on page 529 in your textbook.

1. Why do you think Kelly Brady had blood drawn at 1230 for an AST measurement and a platelet count?

- Click on **Chart** and then **203**.
- Click on **Laboratory Reports**.
- Scroll to the report for Wednesday 1230 to locate the results of these tests.

2. Complete the table below based on your review of the Laboratory Reports and Table 25-2 on page 523 in your textbook.

Test	Wed 1230 Result	Value in Preeclampsia/ HELLP Syndrome
Platelet count		
AST		

- Click on **Return to Nurses' Station**.
- Click on **Patient List**.
- Click on **Get Report** for Kelly Brady.

3. Why has Kelly Brady been transferred to labor and delivery?

4. About half of women with HELLP syndrome also have _____,

although _____ may be absent. HELLP syndrome consists of

_____, _____ enzymes, and _____

count. The prominent symptom of HELLP syndrome is

_____.

Other signs and symptoms include _____, _____, and

_____.

→ • Click on **Return to Nurses' Station.**
• Click on **Chart** and then on **203**.
• Click on **Physician's Notes**.
• Scroll to the note for Wednesday 1530.

5. What is the physician's plan of care for Kelly Brady, in light of the HELLP syndrome diagnosis?

Assume that you will be the nurse caring for Kelly Brady after her surgery while she is receiving magnesium sulfate. Read about this medication on pages 525-529 in your textbook and then answer question 6.

6. All of the assessments/interventions listed below are part of routine nursing care for a patient with severe preeclampsia. Place an X beside the activities that are performed specifically to assess for magnesium toxicity.

_____ Measure/record urine output.

_____ Measure proteinuria using urine dipstick.

_____ Monitor liver enzyme levels and platelet count.

_____ Monitor for headache, visual disturbances, and epigastric pain.

_____ Assess for decreased level of consciousness.

_____ Assess DTRs.

_____ Weigh daily to assess for edema.

_____ Monitor vital signs, especially respiratory rate.

_____ Dim room lights and maintain a quiet environment.

10

Complications of Pregnancy: Hemorrhagic Conditions

👓 **Reading Assignment:** Complications of Pregnancy (Chapter 25, pages 512-518)

Patient: Gabriela Valenzuela, Room 205

Objectives:

- Identify appropriate interventions for managing abruptio placentae.
- Differentiate between the symptoms related to an abruptio placentae compared with those related to a placenta previa.
- Plan and evaluate essential patient education during the acute phase of diagnosis.

Exercise 1

Virtual Hospital Activity

25 minutes

- Sign in to work at Pacific View Regional Hospital on the Obstetrics Floor for Period of Care 1. (*Note*: If you are already in the virtual hospital from a previous exercise, click on **Leave the Floor** and then **Restart the Program** to get to the sign-in window.)
- From the Patient List, select Gabriela Valenzuela.
- Click on **Go to Nurses' Station**.
- Click on **Chart** and then on **205**.
- Click on **Emergency Department**.

1. What transpired that brought Gabriela Valenzuela to the ED? How long had she waited to actually come to the ED? What was the deciding factor in her coming to the ED?

Read about the incidence and etiology of abruptio placentae in your textbook on page 515.

2. Other than a motor vehicle accident, what could result in or increase the risk for having an abruptio placentae?

3. Differential diagnosis is very important when you are confronted with clinical manifestations that could be evidence of more than one process. Based on the information on pages 512-516 of your textbook, compare and contrast abruptio placentae and placenta previa.

Characteristic/Complication	Abruptio Placentae	Placenta Previa
Bleeding		
Shock complication		
Coagulopathy (DIC)		
Uterine tonicity		
Tenderness/pain		
Placenta findings		
Fetal effects		

4. Based on your review of the ED Record, describe the abruption that Gabriela Valenzuela has. Provide supporting documentation from your textbook reading.

 • Click on **Return to Nurses' Station**.
   • Click on **205** at the bottom of the screen.
   • Click on **Patient Care** and then **Nurse-Client Interactions**.
   • Select and view the video titled **0740: Patient Teaching—Fetal Monitoring**. (*Note:* Check the virtual clock to see whether enough time has elapsed. You can use the fast-forward feature to advance the time by 2-minute intervals if the video is not yet available. Then click on **Patient Care** and **Nurse-Client Interactions** to refresh the screen.)

5. Once Gabriela Valenzuela is admitted to the floor, what are her and her husband's concerns? What does the nurse include in her teaching to alleviate those concerns?

• Now select and view the video titled **0805: Patient Teaching—Abruption**. (*Note:* Check the virtual clock to see whether enough time has elapsed. You can use the fast-forward feature to advance the time by 2-minute intervals if the video is not yet available. Then click on **Patient Care** and **Nurse-Client Interactions** to refresh the screen.)

6. According to the video, what will help increase the oxygen supply to the baby and prevent further separation of the placenta?

Exercise 2

Virtual Hospital Activity

20 minutes

- Sign in to work at Pacific View Regional Hospital on the Obstetrics Floor for Period of Care 1. (*Note*: If you are already in the virtual hospital from a previous exercise, click on **Leave the Floor** and then **Restart the Program** to get to the sign-in window.)
- From the Patient List, select Gabriela Valenzuela.
- Click on **Go to Nurses' Station**.

Gabriela Valenzuela is at increased risk for early delivery as a result of the abdominal trauma she suffered and the subsequent occurrence of a grade 1 abruptio placentae. She is currently manifesting signs and symptoms of early labor. According to the Emergency Department notes, she was given a dose of betamethasone and this was to be repeated in 12 hours.

1. What is the purpose of the administration of betamethasone in this patient's scenario? (*Hint*: Review information on pages 585-586 of the textbook.)

- Click on **MAR** and review the betamethasone dosage to be given to Gabriela Valenzuela.
- Click on **Return to Room 205**.
- Click on **Medication Room**.
- Click on **Unit Dosage**.
- Click on drawer **205**.
- Click on **Betamethasone** in the upper left corner of the screen.
- Click on **Put Medication on Tray**.
- Click on **Close Drawer**.
- Click on **View Medication Room**.
- Click on **Preparation**.
- Click on **Prepare** and follow the Preparation Wizard's prompts to complete preparation of Gabriela Valenzuela's betamethasone.
- When the Wizard stops asking questions, click **Finish**.
- Click on **Return to Medication Room**.
- Click on **205** to return to the patient's room.
- Click on **Patient Care**.
- Click on **Medication Administration**.
- Click on **Review Your Medications**.
- Click on the tab marked **Prepared**.

2. According to the text box on the right side of your screen, what is the medication name and dosage that you have prepared for Gabriela Valenzuela?

3. How many mg are you giving to Gabriela Valenzuela based on the answer to the previous question? Is this the correct dosage based on the MAR?

→ • Click on **Return to Room 205**.
  • Click on the **Drug** icon in the lower left corner of the screen.
  • To read about betamethasone, either type the drug name in the search box or scroll through the alphabetic list of medications at the top of the screen.

4. Based on the information provided in the Drug Guide, what is the indication and dosage for pregnant adults?

5. Based on your review of the baseline assessment data in the Drug Guide, what areas need to be assessed in Gabriela Valenzuela's history?

6. Now review the information regarding the administration of this medication. What are three things that need to be taken into consideration when giving this medication in the injection form?

7. What are the rights of medication administration as they relate to the patient?

You are now ready to complete the medication administration.

* Click on **Return to Room 205**.
* Click on **Check Armband**.
* Within the purple box under the patient's photo, find **Betamethasone**. Click the down arrow next to **Select** and choose **Administer**.
* Follow the Medication Wizard's prompts to administer Gabriela Valenzuela's betamethasone. Click **Yes** when asked whether to document the injection in the MAR.
* When the Wizard stops asking questions, click **Finish**.
* Click on **Leave the Floor**.
* Click on **Look at Your Preceptor's Evaluation**.
* Click on **Medication Scorecard** and review the evaluation. How did you do? (*Hint:* For a quick refresher on reading your Medication Scorecard, see the **Getting Started** section of this workbook.)

Exercise 3

Virtual Hospital Activity

20 minutes

* Sign in to work at Pacific View Regional Hospital on the Obstetrics Floor for Period of Care 2. (*Note:* If you are already in the virtual hospital from a previous exercise, click on **Leave the Floor** and then **Restart the Program** to get to the sign-in window.)
* From the Patient List, select Gabriela Valenzuela.
* Click on **Go to Nurses' Station**.
* Click on **Chart** and then **205**.
* Click on **Diagnostic Reports**.

Gabriela Valenzuela had an ultrasound done on Tuesday to determine the source of the bleeding.

1. What were the findings on the ultrasound?

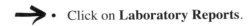 • Click on **Laboratory Reports**.

2. What were Gabriela Valenzuela's hemoglobin and hematocrit levels on Tuesday? How do these compare with Wednesday's report? Has there been a significant change?

 3. According to the textbook information, what other tests need to be performed in preparation for what could happen to these patients? *(Hint:* See pages 516-517 in your textbook.)

 Review pages 515-517 in your textbook.

4. What clinical manifestations would indicate a worsening in the condition of either the patient or the fetus?

 • Click on **Return to Nurses' Station**.
• Click on **EPR**.
• Click on **Login**.
• Select **205** as the patient and **Vital Signs** as the category.
• Using the blue right and left arrows, scroll to review the vital sign findings over the last 12 hours.

5. From 0000 Wednesday until 1200 Wednesday, would you consider Gabriela Valenzuela's condition stable or unstable? State the rationale for your answer.

 • Click on **Exit EPR**.
• Click on **205** at the bottom of the screen.
• Click on **Patient Care** and then **Nurse-Client Interactions**.
• Select and view the video titled **1140: Intervention—Bleeding, Comfort**. (*Note:* Check the virtual clock to see whether enough time has elapsed. You can use the fast-forward feature to advance the time by 2-minute intervals if the video is not yet available. Then click on **Patient Care** and **Nurse-Client Interactions** to refresh the screen.)

6. What happened that elicited this interaction? (*Hint*: Review the Nurse's Notes for Wednesday 1140.)

7. What actions did the nurse take during the interaction?

Exercise 4

Virtual Hospital Activity

15 minutes

- Sign in to work at Pacific View Regional Hospital on the Obstetrics Floor for Period of Care 3. (*Note*: If you are already in the virtual hospital from a previous exercise, click on **Leave the Floor** and then **Restart the Program** to get to the sign-in window.)
- From the Patient List, select Gabriela Valenzuela.
- Click on **Go to Nurses' Station**.
- Click on **Kardex** and then on tab **205**.

1. What problem areas have been identified by the nurse related to Gabriela Valenzuela's diagnosis?

2. What is the focus of the outcomes related to the above-mentioned problems?

3. Using correct NANDA nursing diagnosis terminology, list four possible nursing diagnoses appropriate for Gabriela Valenzuela at this time.

 - Click on **Return to Nurses' Station**.
- Click on **Chart** and then **205**.
- Click on **Patient Education**.

4. According to the Patient Education sheet in Gabriela Valenzuela's chart, what are the educational goals related to the patient's diagnosis?

➡ • Click on **Nurse's Notes**.

5. After reviewing the Nurse's Notes, what education has been completed by the nurses through Period of Care 3? Include the times and topics discussed.

6. What are some barriers to learning that the nurse may confront with this patient?

7. How can the nurse overcome each of these?

Concurrent Disorders During Pregnancy: Gestational Diabetes Mellitus

 Reading Assignment: Concurrent Disorders During Pregnancy
(Chapter 26, pages 536-546)

Patient: Stacey Crider, Room 202

Objectives:

- Identify appropriate interventions for controlling hyperglycemia in a patient with gestational diabetes mellitus (GDM).
- Correctly administer insulin to a patient with GDM.
- Plan and evaluate essential patient teaching for a patient with GDM.

Exercise 1

 Virtual Hospital Activity

🕐 30 minutes

- Sign in to work at Pacific View Regional Hospital on the Obstetrics Floor for Period of Care 2. (*Note*: If you are already in the virtual hospital from a previous exercise, click on **Leave the Floor** and then **Restart the Program** to get to the sign-in window.)
- From the Patient List, select Stacey Crider.
- Click on **Go to Nurses' Station**.
- Click on **Chart** and then **202**.
- Click on **History and Physical**.

1. When was Stacey Crider's GDM diagnosed? How has it been managed thus far?

2. Read about risk factors for GDM on page 541 in your textbook and list them below.

• Search for evidence of risk factors for GDM in Stacey Crider in the **History and Physical** and **Admissions** sections of her chart.

3. Which risk factors for GDM are present in Stacey Crider?

4. What does Stacey Crider's physician suspect is the cause of her poorly controlled blood glucose levels? (*Hint*: See Impression at the end of the History and Physical.)

→ • Click on **Physician's Orders**.

5. Look at Stacey Crider's admission orders. Write down the orders that are related to GDM.

 6. Why did Stacey Crider's physician order a hemoglobin A1C test as part of her admission labs? (*Hint*: See page 539 in your textbook.)

On admission, Stacey Crider was in preterm labor, which was treated with magnesium sulfate tocolysis. She was also given a course of betamethasone.

→ • Click on **Return to Nurses' Station**.
• Click on the **Drug** icon in the lower left corner of the screen.
• Use the Search box or the scroll bar to locate information about betamethasone.

7. How might betamethasone affect Stacey Crider's GDM?

→ • Click on **Return to Nurses' Station**.
• Click on **Chart** and then on **202**.
• Click on **Physician's Notes**.
• Scroll to the note for Tuesday at 0700.

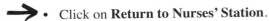

8. How does Stacey Crider's physician plan to deal with these potential medication effects?

Stacey Crider's other admission diagnosis is bacterial vaginosis (BV).

 • Click on **Return to Nurses' Station**.
• Click on **202** at the bottom of your screen.
• Click on **Patient Care** and then on **Nurse-Client Interactions**.
• Select and view the video titled **1115: Teaching—Diet, Infection**. (*Note:* Check the virtual clock to see whether enough time has elapsed. You can use the fast-forward feature to advance the time by 2-minute intervals if the video is not yet available. Then click on **Patient Care** and **Nurse-Client Interactions** to refresh the screen.)

9. What is the relationship between Stacey Crider's bacterial vaginosis infection and her GDM?

Exercise 2

 Virtual Hospital Activity

 20 minutes

• Sign in to work at Pacific View Regional Hospital on the Obstetrics Floor for Period of Care 1. (*Note:* If you are already in the virtual hospital from a previous exercise, click on **Leave the Floor** and then **Restart the Program** to get to the sign-in window.)
• From the Patient List, select Stacey Crider.
• Click on **Go to Nurses' Station**.
• Click on the **Drug** icon in the lower left corner of the screen.
• Scroll down the drug list and click on **Insulin**.

Stacey Crider needs her insulin so that she can eat breakfast. Recall that she receives lispro insulin before each meal and NPH insulin at bedtime. Read about the differences in these two types of insulin in the Drug Guide.

1. Using the information you found in the Drug Guide (specifically the Pharmacokinetics section), complete the table below.

Type of Insulin	Onset of Action	Peak	Duration
Lispro			
NPH			

→ • Click on **EPR** and then on **Login**.
  • Click on **202** in the Patient drop-down menu. Select **Vital Signs** as the category.
  • Look at the vital sign assessment documented on Wednesday at 0700.

2. What is Stacey Crider's blood glucose?

→ • Click on **Exit EPR**.
  • Click on **MAR**.
  • Click on tab **202**.

3. What is Stacey Crider's prescribed insulin dosage?

→ • Click on **Return to Nurses' Station**.
  • Click on **Chart** and then **202**.
  • Click on **Physician's Orders**.
  • Scroll to the orders for Tuesday at 1900.

4. How much insulin should Stacey Crider receive? Why?

→ • Click on **Return to Nurses' Station**.
  • Click on **Medication Room**.
  • Click on **Unit Dosage**.
  • Click on drawer **202**.

- Click on **Insulin Lispro**.
- Click on **Put Medication on Tray**.
- Click on **Close Drawer**.
- Click on **View Medication Room**.
- Click on **Preparation**.
- Click on **Prepare** and follow the prompts to complete preparation of Stacey Crider's lispro insulin dose.
- Click on **Return to Medication Room**.

You are almost ready to give Stacey Crider's insulin injection. However, before you do . . .

5. Considering lispro insulin's rapid onset of action, what else should you check before giving Stacey Crider her injection?

Now you're ready!

- Click on Room **202**.
- Click on **Check Armband**.
- Click on **Patient Care** and then on **Medication Administration**.
- **Insulin Lispro** should be listed on the left side of your screen. Click on the down arrow next to **Select** and choose **Administer**.
- Follow the prompts to administer Stacey Crider's insulin injection. Indicate **Yes** to document the injection in the MAR.
- Click on **Leave the Floor**.
- Click on **Look at Your Preceptor's Evaluation**.
- Click on **Medication Scorecard**. How did you do?

Exercise 3

Virtual Hospital Activity

20 minutes

- Sign in to work at Pacific View Regional Hospital on the Obstetrics Floor for Period of Care 3. (*Note*: If you are already in the virtual hospital from a previous exercise, click on **Leave the Floor** and then **Restart the Program** to get to the sign-in window.)
- From the Patient List, select Stacey Crider.
- Click on **Go to Nurses' Station**.
- Click on **Chart** and then **202**.
- Click on **Patient Education**.

Stacey Crider will likely be discharged home soon. Review her Patient Education record to determine her learning needs in relation to GDM.

1. List the educational goals for Stacey Crider regarding GDM.

Read the section on Application of the Nursing Process: The Pregnant Woman with Diabetes Mellitus on pages 543-546 in your textbook.

2. Which of Stacey Crider's educational goals would apply to all women with GDM?

3. Which of Stacey Crider's educational goals would *not* apply to all women with GDM? Support your answer.

➤ • Click on **Nurse's Notes** and scroll to the note for 0600 Wednesday.

4. How did the nurse describe Stacey Crider's ability to give her own insulin injection at that time?

➤ • Click again on **Patient Education**.

5. What teaching has already been done with this patient on Wednesday in regard to GDM?

➤ • Click on **Nurse's Notes** and scroll to the note for 1200 Wednesday.

6. Do you think today's initial teaching on insulin administration was effective? Support your answer using objective documentation from the nurse's note.

Use the information you have obtained from the Patient Education form and the Nurse's Notes to answer the following questions.

7. Stacey Crider needs to know all of the following information. Which topic(s) would you choose to work on with her during this period of care?

_____ Verbalize appropriate food choices and portions.

_____ Demonstrate good technique when administering insulin.

_____ Demonstrate good technique with self-monitoring of blood glucose.

_____ Recognize hyper- and hypoglycemia and how to treat each.

8. Give a rationale for your answer to question 7.

Read the section on Risk Factors for Gestational Diabetes Mellitus on page 541 in your textbook. Stacey Crider has a significant risk for developing glucose intolerance later in life.

9. What advice would you give Stacey Crider to reduce this risk?

10. Because she has had GDM with this pregnancy, what medical follow-up would you advise for Stacey Crider after her baby is born? Why?

11. Could Stacey Crider's GDM affect her baby after birth? What advice would you give her regarding medical follow-up for her baby?

12 ——————————

Concurrent Disorders During Pregnancy: Selected Infections

————————————————————————————————————

/OO **Reading Assignment:** Concurrent Disorders During Pregnancy
(Chapter 26, pages 556-565)

Patients: Gabriela Valenzuela, Room 205
Laura Wilson, Room 206

Objectives:

- Explain the importance of prophylactic Group B streptococcus treatment.
- Identify risk factors for acquiring HIV infection.
- Prioritize information to be included in patient teaching related to HIV infection.

Exercise 1

 Virtual Hospital Activity

 15 minutes

- Sign in to work at Pacific View Regional Hospital on the Obstetrics Floor for Period of Care 1. (*Note*: If you are already in the virtual hospital from a previous exercise, click on **Leave the Floor** and then **Restart the Program** to get to the sign-in window.)
- From the Patient List, select Gabriela Valenzuela.
- Click on **Go to Nurses' Station**.
- Click on **Chart** and then **205**.
- Click on **History and Physical** and scroll to the plan at the end of this document.

   1. What is the medical plan of care for Gabriela Valenzuela?

2. Is Gabriela Valenzuela known to be positive for Group B streptococcus (GBS)?

 Read about Group B streptococcus infection on page 563 in your textbook; then answer questions 3 through 6.

3. List risk factors for neonatal GBS infection. Which risk factor applies to Gabriela Valenzuela?

4. Since pregnant women with GBS in the vagina are almost always asymptomatic, why does Gabriela Valenzuela need to be treated for this organism?

➡ • Click on **Physician's Orders**.
  • Scroll to the admission orders written Tuesday at 2100.

5. What medication/dosage/frequency will Gabriela Valenzuela receive for Group B strep prophylaxis?

6. How does this order compare with the treatment regimen recommended in your textbook?

Exercise 2

 Virtual Hospital Activity

 35 minutes

- Sign in to work at Pacific View Regional Hospital on the Obstetrics Floor for Period of Care 1. (*Note*: If you are already in the virtual hospital from a previous exercise, click on **Leave the Floor** and then **Restart the Program** to get to the sign-in window.)
- From the Patient List, select Laura Wilson.
- Click on **Go to Nurses' Station**.
- Click on **Chart** and then **206**.
- Click on **Nursing Admission**.

1. What risk factors for acquiring an STI are identified on Laura Wilson's Nursing Admission form?

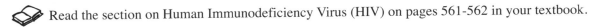 Read the section on Human Immunodeficiency Virus (HIV) on pages 561-562 in your textbook.

2. Currently in the United States, homosexual individuals are more likely than heterosexuals to become infected with HIV.
   a. True
   b. False

➤ • While still in the chart, click on **Admissions**.

3. In the United States today, HIV infection is spreading most rapidly in the groups listed below. Place an X beside the group(s) to which Laura Wilson belongs.

_____   Women

_____   African Americans

_____   Latinos

_____   Women who live in the southern United States

→ • Now click again on **Nursing Admission**.

4. What did the admitting nurse document about Laura Wilson's knowledge and acceptance of her HIV diagnosis?

→ • Click on **Return to Nurses' Station**.
 • Click on **Patient Care** and then **Nurse-Client Interactions**.
 • Select and view the video titled **0800: Teaching—HIV in Pregnancy**. (*Note:* Check the virtual clock to see whether enough time has elapsed. You can use the fast-forward feature to advance the time by 2-minute intervals if the video is not yet available. Then click on **Patient Care** and **Nurse-Client Interactions** to refresh the screen.)

5. Does Laura Wilson appear to be fully aware of the implications of HIV infection? State the rationale for your answer.

6. What coping mechanism is Laura Wilson exhibiting in the video interaction?

→ • Click on **Chart**.
 • Click on **Nursing Admission**.

7. Laura Wilson needs education on all of the following topics. Which would you choose to teach her about at this time?

   _____ Safer sex

   _____ Medication side effects and importance of compliance

   _____ Need for medical follow-up and medication for the baby

   _____ Impact of HIV on birth plans

8. Give a rationale for your answer to question 7.

Concurrent Disorders During Pregnancy: Cardiac/Lupus

 Reading Assignment: Concurrent Disorders During Pregnancy
(Chapter 26, pages 546-551 and 553-555)

Patients: Maggie Gardner, Room 204
Gabriela Valenzuela, Room 205

Objectives:

- Identify appropriate interventions for managing selected medical-surgical problems in pregnancy.
- Plan and evaluate essential patient education during the acute phase of diagnosis.

Exercise 1

 Virtual Hospital Activity

10 minutes

- Sign in to work at Pacific View Regional Hospital on the Obstetrics Floor for Period of Care 1. (*Note*: If you are already in the virtual hospital from a previous exercise, click on **Leave the Floor** and then **Restart the Program** to get to the sign-in window.)
- From the Patient List, select Gabriela Valenzuela.
- Click on **Go to Nurses' Station**.
- Click on **Chart** and then **205**.
- Click on **History and Physical**.

 Review material regarding cardiac problems during pregnancy on pages 546-551 in your textbook.

1. According to the textbook, 1% of pregnancies are complicated with heart disease. In the History and Physical for Gabriela Valenzuela, what does the physician note as her cardiac problem?

2. Mitral valve disease is one of the most common causes of cardiac disease in pregnant women.
   a. True
   b. False

3. According to the History and Physical, what cardiac symptoms does Gabriela Valenzuela exhibit now that she is pregnant?

4. Based on your textbook reading, why do pregnant women with cardiac disorders have problems during their pregnancies?

5. What abnormal assessment finding is noted in the History and Physical that would be associated with Gabriela Valenzuela's cardiac disorder?

Exercise 2

Virtual Hospital Activity

20 minutes

Autoimmune disorders encompass a wide variety of disorders that can be disruptive to the pregnancy process. Maggie Gardner has been admitted to rule out lupus. The following activities will explore the various aspects of this autoimmune disorder. Review the information regarding systemic lupus erythematosus (SLE) on pages 553-555 in your textbook.

- Sign in to work at Pacific View Regional Hospital on the Obstetrics Floor for Period of Care 1. (*Note*: If you are already in the virtual hospital from a previous exercise, click on **Leave the Floor** and then **Restart the Program** to get to the sign-in window.)
- From the Patient List, select Maggie Gardner.
- Click on **Go to Nurses' Station**.
- Click on **Chart** and then **204**.
- Click on **History and Physical**.

1. Based on Maggie Gardner's History and Physical, what information would correlate to a diagnosis of SLE?

2. According to the textbook, what might pose a special risk during pregnancy?

- Click on **Return to Nurses' Station**.
- Click on Room **204** at the bottom of the screen.
- Click on **Patient Care** and then on **Physical Assessment**.
- Click on various body areas (yellow boxes) and system subcategories (green boxes) to perform a head-to-toe assessment of Maggie Gardner.

3. Based on your head-to-toe assessment, list four abnormal findings that are related to Maggie Gardner's diagnosis.

- Click on **Chart** and then on **204**.
- Click on **Patient Education**.

4. Based on your physical assessment, the information from the Patient Education section of the chart, and the fact that this is a new diagnosis for the patient, list three areas of teaching that need to be completed with Maggie Gardner.

Exercise 3

Virtual Hospital Activity

35 minutes

- Sign in to work at Pacific View Regional Hospital on the Obstetrics Floor for Period of Care 3. (*Note*: If you are already in the virtual hospital from a previous exercise, click on **Leave the Floor** and then **Restart the Program** to get to the sign-in window.)
- From the Patient List, select Maggie Gardner.
- Click on **Go to Nurses' Station**.
- Click on **Chart** and then **204**.
- Click on the **Consultations** tab.
- Review the Rheumatology Consult.

1. List four things that the rheumatologist notes in her impressions regarding specific findings that are associated with a diagnosis of SLE for Maggie Gardner.

 • Click on **Diagnostic Reports**.

2. Maggie Gardner had an ultrasound done before the consult with the rheumatologist. What were the findings as they relate to SLE? What were the follow-up recommendations? (*Hint*: See Impressions section.)

3. What is the rheumatologist's plan regarding laboratory/diagnostics to gain a definitive diagnosis?

4. According to the Rheumatology Consult, what is the plan regarding medications (immediate need)?

- Click on **Return to Nurses' Station**.
- Click on the **Drug** icon in the lower left corner of the screen.
- Find the Drug Guide profile of prednisone. (*Hint:* You can type the drug name in the Search box or scroll through the alphabetic list of drugs at the top of the screen.)

5. What does Maggie Gardner need to be taught regarding this medication?

- Click on **Return to Nurses' Station**.
- Click on Room **204**.
- Click on **Patient Care** and then **Nurse-Client Interactions**.
- Select and view the video titled **1530: Disease Management**. (*Note:* Check the virtual clock to see whether enough time has elapsed. You can use the fast-forward feature to advance the time by 2-minute intervals if the video is not yet available. Then click on **Patient Care** and **Nurse-Client Interactions** to refresh the screen.)

6. During this video clip, the nurse provides Maggie Gardner with information regarding her disease. What two things does the nurse note that are important aspects of the patient's disease management during pregnancy?

7. What medication ordered by the rheumatologist will assist in the blood flow to the placenta? How?

8. What key component does the nurse identify for Maggie Gardner that will assist in maintaining a healthy pregnancy?

9. What excuse does Maggie Gardner give for not keeping previous doctor's appointments? (*Hint:* This information is also found in the Nursing Admission in the chart.)

Exercise 4

 Virtual Hospital Activity

 15 minutes

- Sign in to work at Pacific View Regional Hospital on the Obstetrics Floor for Period of Care 4. (*Note*: If you are already in the virtual hospital from a previous exercise, click on **Leave the Floor** and then **Restart the Program** to get to the sign-in window.)
- From the Nurses' Station, click on **Chart** and then **204**. (*Remember:* You are not able to visit patients or administer medications during Period of Care 4. You are able to review patient records only.)
- Click on **Laboratory Reports**.

1. The results are now available for the following laboratory tests that were ordered during Period of Care 2. Record the findings below.

Laboratory Test	Result
C3	
C4	
CH50	
RPR	
ANA Titer	
Anticardiolipin	
Anti-sm; Anti-DNA; Anti-SSA	
Anti-SSB	
Anti-RVV; Antiphospholipid	

 - Click on **Consultations** and review the Rheumatology Consult.

2. The lab findings you recorded in question 1 are definitive for the diagnosis of SLE. According to the textbook and the Rheumatology Consult, what is the plan to manage this disease once the baby is delivered?

➡ • Click on **Nurse's Notes.**

3. By Period of Care 4, Maggie Gardner has been provided with education regarding various aspects of her disease process, testing, and hospital procedures. Based on your review of the Nurse's Notes for Wednesday, what has she been specifically taught? Include the time each instruction took place.

4. Using correct NANDA nursing diagnosis terminology, write three possible nursing diagnoses for Maggie Gardner.

5. SLE requires long-term management because patients will experience remissions and exacerbations. What step did the rheumatologist take with Maggie Gardner to begin the long-term relationship that will be required to ensure a healthy outcome?

Intrapartum Complications

 Reading Assignment: Intrapartum Complications (Chapter 27)

Patients: Dorothy Grant, Room 201
Stacey Crider, Room 202
Kelly Brady, Room 203
Gabriela Valenzuela, Room 205

Objectives:

- Assess and identify signs and symptoms present in the patient experiencing preterm labor.
- Describe appropriate nursing care for the patient in preterm labor.
- Develop a birth plan to meet the needs of the preterm infant.

Exercise 1

 Virtual Hospital Activity

20 minutes

- Sign in to work at Pacific View Regional Hospital on the Obstetrics Floor for Period of Care 2. (*Note*: If you are already in the virtual hospital from a previous exercise, click on **Leave the Floor** and then **Restart the Program** to get to the sign-in window.)
- From the Patient List, select Dorothy Grant and Gabriela Valenzuela.
- Click on **Go to Nurses' Station**.
- Click on **Chart** and then on **201** for Dorothy Grant's chart.
- Click on **History and Physical**.

1. Using the information found in the History and Physical section, complete the table below for Dorothy Grant.

Patient	Weeks Gestation	Reason for Admission
Dorothy Grant		

- Click on **Return to Nurses' Station**.
- Click again on **Chart**; this time, select **205** for Gabriela Valenzuela's chart.
- Click on **History and Physical**.

2. Using the information found in the History and Physical section, complete the table below for Gabriela Valenzuela.

Patient	Weeks Gestation	Reason for Admission
Gabriela Valenzuela		

- Click on **Return to Nurses' Station**.
- Click on **201** at the bottom of the screen to go to Dorothy Grant's room.
- Click on **Patient Care** and then on **Physical Assessment**.
- Click on **Pelvic** and then on **Reproductive**.

3. Complete the table below with the results of Dorothy Grant's initial cervical examination.

Patient	Time	Dilation	Effacement	Station
Dorothy Grant				

- Click on **Return to Nurses' Station**.
- Click on **205** to go to Gabriela Valenzuela's room.
- Click on **Patient Care** and then on **Physical Assessment**.
- Click on **Pelvic** and then on **Reproductive**.

4. Record the results of Gabriela Valenzuela's initial cervical examination in the table below.

Patient	Time	Dilation	Effacement	Station
Gabriela Valenzuela				

Read the definition of preterm labor on page 579 in your textbook.

5. Preterm labor is defined as the onset of labor after the _____

   but before the _____
   of the pregnancy.

6. As of Wednesday at 0800, would you consider both these patients to be in preterm labor? Give a rationale for your answer.

Read the section on Tocolytics on pages 583-585 in your textbook.

7. Match each of the medications below with the description of how it works as a tocolytic agent. (*Hint:* Letters may be used more than once.)

   _____ Magnesium sulfate

   _____ Nifedipine (Procardia)

   _____ Ritodrine (Yutopar)

   _____ Terbutaline (Brethine)

   _____ Indomethacin (Indocin)

   a. Blocks calcium from entering smooth muscle cells, thus relaxing uterine contractions

   b. Inhibits uterine muscle activity as a result of stimulation of beta-adrenergic receptors of the sympathetic nervous system

   c. Exact mechanism unclear, but promotes relaxation of smooth muscles

   d. Suppresses preterm labor by inhibiting the synthesis of prostaglandins

Exercise 2

Virtual Hospital Activity

30 minutes

- Sign in to work at Pacific View Regional Hospital on the Obstetrics Floor for Period of Care 1. (*Note*: If you are already in the virtual hospital from a previous exercise, click on **Leave the Floor** and then **Restart the Program** to get to the sign-in window.)
- From the Patient List, select Stacey Crider.
- Click on **Get Report**.

Stacey Crider was admitted yesterday in preterm labor and put on magnesium sulfate. Her other admission diagnoses were bacterial vaginosis and gestational diabetes with poorly controlled blood glucose levels.

1. What is Stacey Crider's current status in regard to preterm labor?

- Click on **Go to Nurses' Station**.
- Click on **Chart** and then **202**.
- Click on **Physician's Orders**.
- Scroll to the orders for Wednesday at 0715.

2. Which of these orders relate specifically to Stacey Crider's diagnosis of preterm labor?

- Scroll to the orders for Wednesday at 0730.

3. What medication changes are ordered?

Read the drug information on terbutaline on pages 584-585 in your textbook.

4. Why do you think Stacey Crider's physician changed his orders so quickly?

 • Click on **Return to Nurses' Station**.
• Click on **202** at the bottom of the screen.
• Inside the patient's room, click on **Take Vital Signs**.

5. What are Stacey Crider's current vital signs?

Temperature

Heart rate

Respiratory rate

Blood pressure

 6. Which of these parameters provides the most important information you would need before giving Stacey Crider's nifedipine dose? Why? (*Hint*: Read about calcium antagonists on pages 583-585 in your textbook.)

Like Dorothy Grant and Kelly Brady, Stacey Crider is receiving betamethasone.

 Read about Accelerating Fetal Lung Maturity in your textbook on pages 585-586. Also consult the drug guide on betamethasone and dexamethasone on page 586.

7. Why are all three of these patients receiving corticosteroids?

8. What other benefits does this class of medication seem to provide for preterm infants?

→ • Click on **MAR**.
  • Click on tab **202**.

9. What is Stacey Crider's prescribed betamethasone dosage?

10. How does this dosage compare with the recommended dosage listed in your textbook?

→ • Click on **Return to Nurses' Station**.
  • Click on **Medication Room**.
  • Click on **Unit Dosage**.
  • Click on drawer **202**.
  • Click on **Betamethasone**.
  • Click on **Put Medication on Tray**.
  • Click on **Close Drawer**.
  • Click on **View Medication Room**.
  • Click on **Preparation**.
  • Click on **Prepare** and follow the Preparation Wizard's prompts to complete preparation of Stacey Crider's betamethasone dose.
  • Click on **Return to Medication Room**.
  • Click on **202** to return to Stacey Crider's room.
  • Click on **Check Armband**.
  • Click on **Check Allergies**.
  • Click on **Patient Care** and then on **Medication Administration**.
  • Find **Betamethasone** listed on the left side of your screen. To its right, click on the down arrow to **Select** and choose **Administer**.
  • Follow the Administration Wizard's prompts to administer Stacey Crider's betamethasone injection. Indicate **Yes** to document the injection in the MAR.
  • Click on **Leave the Floor**.
  • Click on **Look at Your Preceptor's Evaluation**.
  • Click on **Medication Scorecard**. How did you do?

Exercise 3

 Virtual Hospital Activity

 30 minutes

- Sign in to work at Pacific View Regional Hospital on the Obstetrics Floor for Period of Care 4. (*Note*: If you are already in the virtual hospital from a previous exercise, click on **Leave the Floor** and then **Restart the Program** to get to the sign-in window.)
- Click on **Chart** and then **201**. (*Remember:* You are not able to visit patients or administer medications during Period of Care 4. You are able to review patient records only.)
- Click on **Nurse's Notes**.
- Scroll to the note for Wednesday 1815.

1. What are the findings from Dorothy Grant's cervical examination at this time?

 - Scroll to the note for Wednesday 1840. It states that Dorothy Grant is being prepped for delivery.

 2. If you were the nurse caring for Dorothy Grant during delivery, what special preparations would you make to care for the baby immediately after birth? (*Hint:* Read the section on Teaching What May Occur During a Preterm Birth on page 588 in your textbook.)

 - Click on **Return to Nurses' Station**.
- Click again on **Chart** and then **205** for Gabriela Valenzuela's chart.
- Click on **Physician's Notes**.
- Scroll to the note for Wednesday 0800.

3. What is the anticipated outcome of Gabriela Valenzuela's labor, according to this note?

• Scroll to the notes for Wednesday 1415 and 1455.

4. What preparations have been made during the day for the birth of Gabriela Valenzuela's baby?

 Read the section on Cesarean Birth on pages 374-384 in your textbook.

 • Click on **Return to Nurses' Station**.
• Click on **Chart** and then **203** for Kelly Brady's chart.
• Click on **Physician's Notes**.
• Scroll to the note for Wednesday 1530.

Kelly Brady was admitted yesterday with severe preeclampsia at 26 weeks gestation. Her preeclampsia is now worsening.

5. Why does Kelly Brady's physician now recommend immediate delivery?

6. What general risks related to cesarean section does Kelly Brady's physician discuss with her?

7. Because of Kelly Brady's early gestational age (26 weeks), her physician anticipates a classical uterine incision. How will this type of incision affect Kelly Brady's birth options in future pregnancies?

• Click on **Physician's Orders**.
  • Scroll to the orders for Wednesday 1540.

8. List the orders to be carried out before Kelly Brady's surgery. State the purpose of each.

Order	Purpose

9. Can you think of other common preoperative procedures? List them below. (*Hint*: Refer to a basic Medical-Surgical textbook for ideas if you need help!)

LESSON 15

High-Risk Newborns

Reading Assignment: The Childbearing Family with Special Needs (Chapter 24)
Concurrent Disorders During Pregnancy (Chapter 26)
High-Risk Newborn: Complications Associated with
Gestational Age and Development (Chapter 29)
High-Risk Newborn: Acquired and Congenital Conditions
(Chapter 30)

Patients: Stacey Crider, Room 202
Kelly Brady, Room 203
Gabriela Valenzuela, Room 205
Laura Wilson, Room 206

Objectives:

- Describe commonly occurring problems of infants of diabetic mothers.
- List nursing interventions related to hypoglycemia in infants of diabetic mothers.
- Identify risk factors for development of early-onset Group B strep infection and HIV infection.
- Describe common signs and symptoms of early-onset Group B strep infection.
- List nursing interventions for preventing transmission of the HIV virus to the neonate.
- Identify signs and symptoms of in utero drug exposure in the neonate.
- Identify common problems found in extremely low-birth-weight infants.

Exercise 1

 Virtual Hospital Activity

 20 minutes

- Sign in to work at Pacific View Regional Hospital on the Obstetrics Floor for Period of Care 4. (*Note*: If you are already in the virtual hospital from a previous exercise, click on **Leave the Floor** and then **Restart the Program** to get to the sign-in window.)
- Click on **Chart** and then on **202** for Stacey Crider's chart. (*Remember:* You are not able to visit patients or administer medications during Period of Care 4. You are able to review patient records only.)
- Click on **History and Physical**.
- Scroll to History of Present Illness.

1. When was Stacey Crider's gestational diabetes diagnosed?

2. How was Stacey Crider's gestational diabetes managed?

 • Click on **Nursing Admission** and scroll to Diagnosis.

3. What was the status of Stacey Crider's gestational diabetes when she was admitted to the hospital at 27 weeks gestation?

Assume that Stacey Crider has given birth and you are now the nurse caring for her baby. Refer to Table 26-1 on page 538 and read pages 538-540 and pages 664-665 in your textbook.

4. Listed below are problems often seen in infants of diabetic mothers. Match each problem with the mechanism(s) responsible for that complication. (*Hint:* Letters may be used more than once.)

_____ Congenital anomalies

_____ Macrosomia

_____ Hypoglycemia

_____ Small-for-gestational-age (SGA) infant

_____ Respiratory distress syndrome

_____ Polycythemia

a. Hyperglycemia

b. Maternal severe vascular disease

c. High fetal insulin levels

5. The most frequent sign of low glucose is _____.

Other common signs of hypoglycemia include _____,

_____, _____, and _____.

Glucose levels reach their lowest point at _____ after birth.

6. List three nursing interventions to prevent or manage hypoglycemia in Stacey Crider's baby.

Exercise 2

 Virtual Hospital Activity

 30 minutes

Gabriela Valenzuela was admitted at 34 weeks gestation with vaginal bleeding and uterine contractions following an MVA. Her labor progressed throughout the day on Wednesday, and vaginal delivery is expected.

- Sign in to work at Pacific View Regional Hospital on the Obstetrics Floor for Period of Care 4. (*Note*: If you are already in the virtual hospital from a previous exercise, click on **Leave the Floor** and then **Restart the Program** to get to the sign-in window.)
- Click on **MAR**, and then on tab **205** for Gabriela Valenzuela's records. (*Remember:* You are not able to visit patients or administer medications during Period of Care 4. You are able to review patient records only.)

1. What medication has Gabriela Valenzuela been receiving today for Group B streptococcus prophylaxis?

➜ • Click on **Return to Nurses' Station**.
- Click on **Chart** and then **205**.
- Click on **Nurse's Notes**.
- Scroll to the note for Wednesday 1820.

2. What are the findings of Gabriela Valenzuela's cervical exam at this time?

 Assume that Gabriela Valenzuela does give birth today. Read the section on Group B Streptococcus Infection on page 563 in your textbook.

3. All of the following are risk factors for the development of early-onset GBS infection. Place an X beside the risk factor that you know would apply to Gabriela Valenzuela's baby.

_____ Preterm birth

_____ Rupture of membranes of more than 18 hours

_____ Maternal fever

_____ Previous infant with GBS infection

4. Some common causes of neonatal sepsis currently are Group _____

   and _____. Early-onset sepsis is usually acquired

   _____, often from complications of labor such as

   _____, _____, or

   _____.

5. If you were the nurse caring for Gabriela Valenzuela's baby, what signs/symptoms might you see if the baby developed early-onset GBS? (*Hint:* See Table 30-1 on pages 661-662 of your textbook.)

Laura Wilson is a G1 P0 at 37 weeks gestation who is also HIV-positive. She was admitted last night with fever, vomiting, and diarrhea to rule out acute abdomen and pyelonephritis. During the day on Wednesday, Laura Wilson began having mild uterine contractions.

→ • From the Nurses' Station, click on **Chart** and then **206**.
  • Click on **Physician's Notes**.
  • Scroll to the note for Wednesday at 0830.

6. Below, record Laura Wilson's HIV-related lab values.

CD4 count

HIV-1 RNA count

→ • Click on **Physician's Orders**.
  • Scroll to the admission orders for Tuesday at 2130.

7. What is Laura Wilson's current antiretroviral drug regimen?

→ • Click on **Nurse's Notes**.
  • Scroll to the note for Wednesday 1830.

8. What event occurred at 1815?

9. Is Laura Wilson in labor at this time? Support your answer.

Laura Wilson is transferred to labor and delivery to give birth. Assume that she does give birth today. Read the section on Human Immunodeficiency Virus on pages 561-562 in your textbook.

10. List factors that, if present, would increase the risk for transmission of HIV from Laura Wilson to her baby during the birth process.

11. Which risk factor does Laura Wilson have at this time?

Refer to Table 30-1 on pages 661-662 in your textbook to answer questions 12-14.

12. Assume that you are the nurse caring for Laura Wilson's baby in the newborn nursery. List nursing interventions to decrease the risk for viral transmission to the baby.

13. If Laura Wilson's baby does become infected with the HIV virus, when would you expect signs of the illness to become apparent?

14. List common signs of HIV infection in infants.

Exercise 3

Virtual Hospital Activity

15 minutes

In addition to being HIV-positive, Laura Wilson also has a past and current history of substance abuse.

- Sign in to work at Pacific View Regional Hospital on the Obstetrics Floor for Period of Care 4. (*Note*: If you are already in the virtual hospital from a previous exercise, click on **Leave the Floor** and then **Restart the Program** to get to the sign-in window.)
- Click on **Chart** and then on **206** for Laura Wilson's chart. (*Remember:* You are not able to visit patients or administer medications during Period of Care 4. You are able to review patient records only.)
- Click on **Nursing Admission**.

1. Complete the chart below with information on Laura Wilson's current use of alcohol and recreational drugs (found on page 4 of the Nursing Admission).

Substance	Reported Use
Alcohol	
Marijuana	
Crack cocaine	

Read about the neonatal effects of tobacco, alcohol, marijuana, and cocaine in the Substance Abuse section on pages 486-488 in your textbook.

2. Listed below and on the next page are problems often seen in infants exposed prenatally to tobacco, alcohol, marijuana, or cocaine. Indicate the substance(s) thought to be associated with each problem by marking an X in the proper column(s). (*Note:* More than one drug may be associated with each problem.)

Problem	Tobacco	Alcohol	Marijuana	Cocaine
Facial anomalies				
Decreased birth weight				
Hyperactivity				
Sudden infant death syndrome (SIDS) or fetal demise				
Congenital abnormalities				
Developmental delay				
Hyperirritability and tremors				
Tachycardia				
Neurobehavioral problems				
Difficult to console				
Prematurity				

 Read the section on Nursing Considerations on pages 666-669 in your textbook. A common nursing diagnosis for parents of drug-exposed infants is Impaired parenting related to lack of understanding of the infant's characteristics and how to relate to him or her.

3. Assume that you are the nurse assigned to work with Laura Wilson and her newborn. List several appropriate nursing interventions to promote parental attachment.

Exercise 4

 Virtual Hospital Activity

 20 minutes

Kelly Brady was admitted with severe preeclampsia at 26 weeks gestation. Because of worsening maternal condition, she gives birth on Wednesday by cesarean section.

- Sign in to work at Pacific View Regional Hospital on the Obstetrics Floor for Period of Care 4. (*Note*: If you are already in the virtual hospital from a previous exercise, click on **Leave the Floor** and then **Restart the Program** to get to the sign-in window.)
- Click on **Chart** and then on **203** for Kelly Brady's chart. (*Remember:* You are not able to visit patients or administer medications during Period of Care 4. You are able to review patient records only.)
- Click on **Diagnostic Reports**.

1. According to the ultrasound done on Tuesday, what is Kelly Brady's baby's estimated fetal weight?

 - Click on **Consultations**.
- Review the Neonatology Consult for Wednesday at 0800.

2. List common problems for babies born at 26 weeks gestation at Pacific View Regional Hospital, according to the neonatologist who met with Kelly Brady and her husband.

 Read the definitions related to birth weight categories found on pages 621-623 and 646-647 in your textbook.

3. If Kelly Brady's baby's actual birth weight is close to her estimated weight, in which weight category will she be placed? Why?

Read the section on Assessment and Care of Common Problems (pages 623-628) in your textbook.

4. The preterm infant is at risk for a number of problems and complications. In the list below, place an X beside the problems that were specifically addressed by the neonatologist during his consultation with Kelly Brady. (*Hint:* See your answer to question 2.)

_____ Thermoregulation

_____ Fluid and electrolyte balance

_____ Skin problems

_____ Infection

_____ Pain

_____ Respiratory distress syndrome

_____ Transient tachypnea of newborn

_____ Periventricular-intraventricular hemorrhage

_____ Retinopathy of prematurity

_____ Necrotizing enterocolitis

5. Write a nursing diagnosis appropriate for Kelly Brady and her husband, as parents of a premature baby who will have an extended NICU stay.

6. List several nursing interventions to assist the Bradys in assuming their role as parents.

LESSON **16** ———————————————

Reproductive System Concerns, Contraception, and Infertility

Reading Assignment: Reproductive Anatomy and Physiology (Chapter 4)
Family Planning (Chapter 31)
Infertility (Chapter 32)

Patients: Stacey Crider, Room 202
Kelly Brady, Room 203
Maggie Gardner, Room 204
Gabriela Valenzuela, Room 205
Laura Wilson, Room 206

Objectives:

- Identify reproductive issues that can occur.
- Differentiate between the varying types of contraception available.
- Identify various methods of testing and treatment options that can be used for couples experiencing infertility concerns.

Exercise 1

 Virtual Hospital Activity

 10 minutes

 Review pages 44-45 and 51-53 in your textbook.

1. What is a normal length for a menstrual cycle?

2. What are the criteria to diagnose an individual with primary amenorrhea? Secondary amenorrhea?

 • Sign in to work at Pacific View Regional Hospital on the Obstetrics Floor for Period of Care 1. (*Note*: If you are already in the virtual hospital from a previous exercise, click on **Leave the Floor** and then **Restart the Program** to get to the sign-in window.)
• From the Patient List, select Stacey Crider.
• Click on **Go to Nurses' Station**.
• Click on **Chart** and then on **202**.
• Click on **History and Physical**.
• Review the patient's gynecologic history.

3. Does Stacey Crider meet the textbook criteria for amenorrhea?

4. What is her history?

5. List three things that can cause amenorrhea.

Exercise 2

 Virtual Hospital Activity

 20 minutes

 Review pages 679-699 in your textbook.

1. What is family planning?

2. No form of contraceptive is 100% effective in preventing _____.

 • Sign in to work at Pacific View Regional Hospital on the Obstetrics Floor for Period of Care 1. (*Note*: If you are already in the virtual hospital from a previous exercise, click on **Leave the Floor** and then **Restart the Program** to get to the sign-in window.)
   • From the Patient List, select Kelly Brady, Gabriela Valenzuela, and Laura Wilson.
   • Click on **Go to Nurses' Station**.
   • Click on **Chart** and then on **203** for Kelly Brady's chart.
   • Review the **History and Physical**.
   • Repeat the previous two steps for Gabriela Valenzuela and Laura Wilson.

3. Based on your review of the charts, list the birth control method each of these women was using before her current pregnancy.

Kelly Brady

Gabriela Valenzuela

Laura Wilson

4. When a nurse is assisting individuals with contraception, what topics need to be reviewed?

5. Given that Gabriela Valenzuela is Catholic, which method of birth control would be appropriate for the nurse to discuss with her?

6. What does this method rely on?

Review pages 686-699 in your textbook; then answer questions 7 and 8.

7. Kelly Brady wants to use oral contraceptives while breastfeeding to prevent pregnancy. Which type of oral contraception is appropriate for her to use? Why?

8. Laura Wilson is HIV-positive. What is the most appropriate form of birth control for her? Why?

Exercise 3

Virtual Hospital Activity

20 minutes

Review Chapter 32 in your textbook.

1. _____ couples of the reproductive age population has a problem with infertility.

2. Women in their _____ have an increased incidence of infertility.

Maggie Gardner is 41 years old. Let's consider some of the options she had while attempting to get pregnant.

3. List factors that affect male fertility. (*Hint:* Review subheadings in chapter.)

4. List factors that affect female fertility.

 • Sign in to work at Pacific View Regional Hospital on the Obstetrics Floor for Period of
   Care 1. (*Note*: If you are already in the virtual hospital from a previous exercise, click on
   Leave the Floor and then **Restart the Program** to get to the sign-in window.)
 • From the Patient List, select Maggie Gardner.
 • Click on **Go to Nurses' Station**.
 • Click on **Chart** and then on **204**.
 • Review the **History and Physical**.

5. Maggie Gardner was married _____ years before conceiving the first time.

6. Based on the textbook reading, which of the following would Maggie Gardner have been
   diagnosed with if she had chosen to get treatment after a year of attempting to get pregnant?
   a. Primary infertility
   b. Secondary infertility

 Review Table 32-1 on page 703 in your textbook to answer the following questions.

7. What tests can be completed on a female patient to determine the causes of infertility?

8. What tests can be completed on a male patient to determine the causes of infertility?

9. What test is used to assess a couple to determine adequacy of coital technique?

10. What therapies are available to assist an infertile couple in conceiving?

11. What methods did Maggie Gardner and her husband use to assist in getting pregnant? (*Hint*: Review the OB history in the History and Physical.)

Medication Administration

Patients: Dorothy Grant, Room 201
Stacey Crider, Room 202
Maggie Gardner, Room 204
Laura Wilson, Room 206

Objective:

- Correctly administer selected medications to obstetric patients, observing the rights of medication administration.

Exercise 1

 Virtual Hospital Activity

 30 minutes

Dorothy Grant was admitted at 30 weeks gestation for observation following blunt abdominal trauma (she was kicked in the abdomen). She is bleeding vaginally and may have sustained a placental abruption. Your assignment for this exercise is to give Rho(D) immune globulin to Dorothy Grant.

- Sign in to work at Pacific View Regional Hospital on the Obstetrics Floor for Period of Care 2. (*Note*: If you are already in the virtual hospital from a previous exercise, click on **Leave the Floor** and then **Restart the Program** to get to the sign-in window.)
- From the Patient List, select Dorothy Grant.

 Read about Rho(D) immune globulin on page 532 in your textbook.

1. Rho(D) immune globulin is given to prevent production of _____

in Rh-_____ women who have been exposed to Rh-_____ blood

by _____.

169

2. All of the following are reasons that Rho(D) immune globulin might be administered. Place an X next to the reason it has been ordered for Dorothy Grant.

_____   Within 72 hours of giving birth to an Rh-positive infant

_____   Prophylactically at 28 weeks gestation

_____   Following an incident or exposure risk that occurs after 28 weeks gestation

_____   During first trimester pregnancy following miscarriage or elective abortion or ectopic pregnancy

3. List the information about Dorothy Grant that must be determined before giving her Rho(D) immune globulin.

➤ • Click on **Go to Nurses' Station**.
   • Click on **Chart** and then on **201**.
   • Click on **Physician's Orders**.
   • Scroll to the orders for Wednesday 0730.

4. Write the physician's order for Rho(D) immune globulin.

5. According to your textbook, is this the correct dosage and route?

➤ • Click on **Laboratory Reports**.
   • Locate the results for 0245 Wednesday.
   • Scroll down to find the type and screen results.

6. Dorothy Grant's blood type is _____.

7. What additional information do you need? Why? Is that information available?

 • Click on **Return to Nurses' Station**.
- Click on **Medication Room**.
- Click on **Refrigerator**; then click on the refrigerator door to open it.
- Click on **Put Medication on Tray**.
- Click on **Close Door**.
- Click on **View Medication Room**.
- Click on **Preparation**.
- Click on **Prepare** and follow the prompts to complete preparation of this medication.
- Click on **Return to Medication Room**.
- Click on **201** to go to Dorothy Grant's room.
- Click on **Check Armband**.
- Click on **Patient Care**.
- Click on **Medication Administration**.

You are almost ready to give Dorothy Grant's injection. However, before you do . . .

8. Rho(D) immune globulin is often considered a blood product.
   a. True
   b. False

9. Suppose Dorothy Grant absolutely refuses to accept blood or blood products because of her religious beliefs. How would you handle the situation?

Now you're ready to administer the medication!

- Click on the down arrow next to **Select**; choose **Administer**.
- Follow the prompts to administer Dorothy Grant's injection. Indicate **Yes** to document the injection in the MAR.
- Click on **Leave the Floor**.
- Click on **Look at Your Preceptor's Evaluation**.
- Click on **Medication Scorecard**. How did you do?

Exercise 2

 Virtual Hospital Activity

 20 minutes

- Sign in to work at Pacific View Regional Hospital on the Obstetrics Floor for Period of Care 1. (*Note*: If you are already in the virtual hospital from a previous exercise, click on **Leave the Floor** and then **Restart the Program** to get to the sign-in window.)
- From the Patient List, select Maggie Gardner.
- Click on **Go to Nurses' Station**.
- Click on the **Chart** and then on **204**.
- Click on the **Nursing Admission**.

1. Maggie Gardner verbalizes anxiety repeatedly throughout the Nursing Admission. What is her primary concern? Why? Provide documentation.

2. Maggie Gardner states that before this pregnancy she had a highly adaptive coping mechanism. How does she consider her ability to cope at this point? Why? (*Hint*: See the Coping and Stress Tolerance section in the Nursing Admission.)

➤ • Click on the **Physician's Orders**.

   3. What medication has the physician ordered to help Maggie Gardner with her anxiety?

➤ • Click on **Return to Nurses' Station**.
  • Click on the **Drug** icon in the lower left corner of your screen.
  • Use the Search box or the scroll bar to find the medication you identified in question 3.
  • Review all of the information provided regarding this drug.

   4. What is the drug's mechanism of action?

➤ • Click on **Return to Nurses' Station**.
  • Click on **204** to go to Maggie Gardner's room.
  • Click on **Patient Care** and then **Nurse-Client Interactions**.
  • Select and view the video titled **0745: Evaluation—Efficacy of Drugs**. (*Note:* Check the virtual clock to see whether enough time has elapsed. You can use the fast-forward feature to advance the time by 2-minute intervals if the video is not yet available. Then click on **Patient Care** and **Nurse-Client Interactions** to refresh the screen.)

   5. According to the nurse, how long will it take for Maggie Gardner to see therapeutic effects? How does this correlate with what you learned in the Teaching section of the Drug Guide?

Exercise 3

 Virtual Hospital Activity

 15 minutes

In this exercise, you will administer betamethasone to Stacey Crider, who was admitted to the hospital at 27 weeks gestation in preterm labor.

- Sign in to work at Pacific View Regional Hospital on the Obstetrics Floor for Period of Care 1. (*Note*: If you are already in the virtual hospital from a previous exercise, click on **Leave the Floor** and then **Restart the Program** to get to the sign-in window.)
- From the Patient List, select Stacey Crider.

1. Before preparing Stacey Crider's betamethasone, what do you need to do first?

- Click on **Go to Nurses' Station**.
- Click on **Chart** and then **202**.
- Click on **Physician's Orders**.
- Scroll until you find the order for betamethasone.

2. After verifying the physician's order, what is your next step?

- Click on **Return to Nurses' Station**.
- Click on **Medication Room**.
- Click on **Unit Dosage**.
- Click on drawer **202**.
- Click on **Betamethasone**.
- Click on **Put Medication on Tray**.
- Click on **Close Drawer**.
- Click on **View Medication Room**.
- Click on **Preparation**.
- Click on **Prepare** and follow the prompts to complete preparation of Stacey Crider's betamethasone dose.
- Click on **Return to Medication Room**.

3. Now that the medication is prepared, what is your next step?

- Click on **202** to go to the patient's room.
- Click on **Check Armband**.
- Click on **Check Allergies**.
- Click on **Patient Care** and then on **Medication Administration**.
- Click on the down arrow next to **Select** and choose **Administer**.
- Follow the prompts to administer Stacey Crider's betamethasone injection.

4. What is the final step in the process?

- If you haven't already done so, indicate **Yes** to document the injection in the MAR.
- Click on **Leave the Floor**.
- Click on **Look at Your Preceptor's Evaluation**.
- Click on **Medication Scorecard**. How did you do?

Exercise 4

 Virtual Hospital Activity

 30 minutes

- Sign in to work at Pacific View Regional Hospital on the Obstetrics Floor for Period of Care 1. (*Note*: If you are already in the virtual hospital from a previous exercise, click on **Leave the Floor** and then **Restart the Program** to get to the sign-in window.)
- From the Patient List, select Laura Wilson.
- Click on **Go to Nurses' Station**.
- Click on **MAR**.
- Click on the tab for Room **206**.

1. Laura Wilson's medications for Wednesday include several different types of drugs. In the list below, place an X next to the one that is used to treat her HIV-positive status.

   _____ Zidovudine 200 mg PO every 8 hours

   _____ Prenatal multivitamin 1 tablet PO daily

   _____ Lactated Ringer's 75 mL/hr IV continuous

→ • Click on **Return to Nurses' Station**.
   • Click on the **Drug** icon in the lower left corner of the screen.
   • Using the Search box or the scroll bar, find the drug you identified in question 1.

2. What is the drug's mechanism of action?

3. What is the drug's therapeutic effect?

4. Does this medication cross the placenta? Is it distributed in breast milk?

5. What symptoms/side effects of this medication need to be reported to the physician?

6. How should this medication be taken?

7. Your final assignment is to give Laura Wilson the medication that is due at 0800. During these lessons, we have provided you with detailed instructions on how to give medications. Now it is time for you to fly solo. Do not forget the rights of medication administration . . . and have fun!! Document below how you did.

If you would like to get more practice, there are other medications that can be given at the beginning of the first three periods of care. Below is a list of the patients, the medications, the routes of administration, and the administration times you can use. As you practice, be sure to select the correct patient when you sign in. That way, you can get a Medication Scorecard for evaluation after you prepare and administer a medication. (*Remember:* If you need help at any time, refer to the **Getting Started** section of this workbook.)

PERIOD OF CARE 1

Room 201, Dorothy Grant

0730/0800—Betamethasone 12 mg IM

Prenatal multivitamin PO

Room 202, Stacey Crider

0800—Prenatal multivitamin PO

Metronidazole 500 mg PO

Betamethasone 12 mg IM

Insulin lispro Sub-Q

Nifedipine 20 mg PO

Room 203, Kelly Brady

0730/0800—Prenatal multivitamin PO

Ferrous sulfate PO

Labetalol hydrochloride 400 mg PO

Nifedipine 10 mg PO

Room 204, Maggie Gardner

0800—Prenatal multivitamin PO

Buspirone hydrochloride 7.5 mg PO

Room 205, Gabriela Valenzuela

0800—Ampicillin 2 g IV

Betamethasone 12 mg IM

Prenatal multivitamin PO

Room 206, Laura Wilson

0800—Zidovudine 200 mg PO

Prenatal multivitamin PO

PERIOD OF CARE 2

Room 201, Dorothy Grant

1200—Rho(D) immune globulin IM

Room 202, Stacey Crider

1200—Insulin lispro Sub-Q

Room 203, Kelly Brady

1130—Betamethasone 12 mg IM

Room 204, Maggie Gardner

1115—Prednisone 40 mg PO

Aspirin 81 mg PO

PERIOD OF CARE 3

Room 204, Maggie Gardner

1500—Buspirone hydrochloride 7.5 mg PO